INTERNATIONAL VIEWS ON DISABILITY MEASURES: MOVING TOWARD COMPARATIVE MEASUREMENT

RESEARCH IN SOCIAL SCIENCE AND DISABILITY

Series Editors: Sharon N. Barnartt and
Barbara M. Altman

Recent Volumes:

Volume 1: Expanding the Scope of Social Science Research on Disability, Edited by Barbara M. Altman and Sharon N. Barnartt, 2000

Volume 2: Exploring Theories and Expanding Methodologies: Where We Are and Where We Need to Go, Edited by Sharon N. Barnartt and Barbara M. Altman, 2001

Volume 3: Using Survey Data to Study Disability: Results from the National Health Interview Survey on Disability, Edited by Barbara M. Altman, Sharon N. Barnartt, Gerry E. Hendershot, and Sheryl A. Larson, 2003

RESEARCH IN SOCIAL SCIENCE AND DISABILITY
VOLUME 4

INTERNATIONAL VIEWS ON DISABILITY MEASURES: MOVING TOWARD COMPARATIVE MEASUREMENT

EDITED BY

BARBARA M. ALTMAN
National Center for Health Statistics, Hyattsville, Maryland, USA

SHARON N. BARNARTT
Gallaudet University, Washington, DC, USA

Emerald

United Kingdom – North America – Japan
India – Malaysia – China

Emerald Group Publishing Limited
Howard House, Wagon Lane, Bingley BD16 1WA, UK

Reprints and permission service
Contact: booksandseries@emeraldinsight.com

British Library Cataloguing in Publication Data
A catalogue record for this book is available from the British Library

ISBN: 978-0-7623-1282-5
ISSN: 1479-3547 (Series)

Transferred to digital printing 2006

CONTENTS

INTRODUCTION: MEASURING DISABILITY IN THE INTERNATIONAL COMMUNITY
Barbara M. Altman *1*

SECTION I: BACKGROUND

THE WASHINGTON GROUP: ORIGIN AND PURPOSE
Barbara M. Altman *9*

SURVEY MEASUREMENT OF DISABILITY: A REVIEW OF INTERNATIONAL ACTIVITIES AND RECOMMENDATIONS
Gerry E. Hendershot *17*

CULTURAL BELIEFS AND PRACTICES THAT INFLUENCE THE TYPE AND NATURE OF DATA COLLECTED ON INDIVIDUALS WITH DISABILITY THROUGH NATIONAL CENSUS
Nora Groce *41*

REFLECTIONS ON DISABILITY LANGUAGE AND THE ICIDH/ICF
Yerker Andersson *55*

SECTION II: COUNTRY SPECIFIC EXPERIENCES

REVIEW OF PRACTICES IN LESS DEVELOPED COUNTRIES ON THE COLLECTION OF DISABILITY DATA
Angela Me and Margaret Mbogoni *63*

PRODUCTION, DISSEMINATION AND UTILIZATION OF DISABILITY STATISTICS IN UGANDA
Helen Namirembe-Nviiri 89

PARADIGMS LOST: THE CHANGING FACE OF DISABILITY IN RESEARCH
Mitchell E. Loeb and Arne H. Eide 111

PEOPLE WITH DISABILITY IN BRAZIL: A LOOK AT 2000 CENSUS RESULTS
Alicia Bercovich 131

MONITORING PEOPLE WITH DISABILITIES: THE ITALIAN EXPERIENCE
Roberta Crialesi and Elena De Palma 159

SECTION III: METHODOLOGICAL ISSUES

TESTING A DISABILITY QUESTION FOR THE CENSUS
Ken Black 179

PARTICIPATION AND ENVIRONMENT: OUT OF THE MELTING POT AND INTO...?
Ros Madden 225

THE IMPACT OF ASSISTIVE DEVICE USE ON DISABILITY MEASUREMENT
Elizabeth K. Rasch, Barbara M. Altman and Jennifer H. Madans 247

DISABILITY MEASUREMENT MATRIX: A TOOL FOR THE COORDINATION OF MEASUREMENT PURPOSE AND INSTRUMENT DEVELOPMENT
Barbara M. Altman, Elizabeth K. Rasch and Jennifer H. Madans 263

ABOUT THE AUTHORS 285

INTRODUCTION: MEASURING DISABILITY IN THE INTERNATIONAL COMMUNITY

Barbara M. Altman

Disability policy has become an important issue not just in the United States and other developed countries, but around the world from Lesothos to Vietnam and Panama to Palestine. Wars, civil conflicts, natural disasters and environmental poisons along with the effects of normal aging, accidents and poverty have combined to make the worldwide population with disabilities ever growing public health and civil rights issues (Lollar, 2001; Ingstad, 2001). In order to develop and implement policy, nations need to know the size and make-up of their populations who experience disability. Data collected by the Statistical Division of the United Nations over the years has demonstrated how unavailable or inconsistent the data on this population has been over the years. In a preliminary effort to improve the available information and to make it somewhat comparable, the Statistics Division of the Department of Economic and Social Affairs of the U.N. published *Guidelines and Principles for the Development of Disability Statistics* in 2001. The report was prepared in response to activities that had started much earlier, particularly the World Programme of Action concerning disabled persons, which was adopted by the General Assembly in resolution 37/52 on December 3, 1982. Both are major outcomes of the International Year of Disabled Persons.

In addition to the publication of the *Guidelines* in 2001, the United Nations Statistical Division (UNSD) also sponsored a meeting of international

International Views on Disability Measures: Moving Toward Comparative Measurement
Research in Social Science and Disability, Volume 4, 1–6

ISSN: 1479-3547/doi:10.1016/S1479-3547(05)04001-7

experts on measurement of disability in June of that year. As a result of that meeting the Washington Group on Disability Statistics was formed (see Chapter 2 for a more detailed description of the origin of the Washington Group). These complimentary activities were part of a strategy to implement the World Programme of Action, whose purposes are to enhance disability prevention, rehabilitation and equalization of opportunities. Accomplishment of these purposes requires reliable and valid data for planning of policy actions and development of programs. The activities of the Washington Group were expected to provide guidance in development of comparable measures for these purposes.

When this volume is published, the Washington Group will have held its 5th annual meeting where reports will have been made about the basic set of census questions that have been developed and the preparations for pretesting of those questions in national settings around the world. If the pretests show that the questions are workable and comparable, the first major product of the Washington Group will be recommended worldwide for use in national censuses.

Preliminary to getting to this point, however, the initial UNSD meeting and the early Washington Group meetings provided valuable information on the evolution of measurement of disability and the valuable advances in the field. The papers included in this volume are a sampling of the work of the preliminary conference that initiated the activities of the Washington Group as well as a selection of the work presented at the first two meetings of the Washington Group.

IN THIS VOLUME

This volume is divided into three sections providing: information about the background of the development of this international effort to develop culturally compatible measures of disability for use worldwide; examples of what kind of measures are currently in place in a variety of countries; and finally, some examples of the exciting methodological work that is underway to improve measurement and provide the ability to make comparisons cross-nationally.

Background Information

Among the papers in this section is a description of the origin of the Washington Group, which was organized under the auspices of the United

Nations, and is providing the leadership in this quest to improve measurement of disability and provide measures that are culturally comparable. This chapter also provides information about the purpose and objectives of the Washington Group as well as describing its organization and providing the website where more detailed material on its activities can be found.

Chapter 3, contributed by Gerry Hendershot, provides detailed information about the activities and recommendations of other international and supranational organizations around the area of disability measurement. Dr. Hendershot has closely examined the activities of six such organizations reviewing and commenting on the work of each group and providing references to their reports. He gives the first introduction in this volume to the World Health Organization's International Classification of Functioning, Disability and Health (ICF) and uses it as the point of comparison for the recommendations of the international groups he examines.

Other background material is provided through the work of Yerker Andersson and that of Nora Groce. Dr. Groce gives an essential description of the contextual elements that influence how disability is defined in the various cultural settings and how the cultural setting itself can impede or facilitate the collection of the necessary data. An important point that she makes is that while attitudes toward and about disability will impact on the kind of data that will be produced, the understanding of how the data will be used can complicate the data collection process as well. Her work helps us understand why even when there is international agreement on a classification system for disability or on a set of measures to be used in censuses across countries, the results may not be comparable or even compatible.

Dr. Andersson, a former President of the World Federation of the Deaf, provides a view of the measurement issues from the disabled community. He notes the improvement of the ICF over the International Classification of Impairment, Disability and Handicap (ICIDH) and endorses the ICF as a valuable starting point for the measurement process, although he acknowledges some of its limitations as they relate to hearing limitations and possibly in other areas as well.

Country-Specific Experiences

In the second section of the volume some very interesting information is provided on the current uses of measures in a wide variety of areas across the globe. Angela Me and Margaret Mbogoni, using data gathered by the statistical office at the U.N., document the wide variety of approaches by individual countries to identify persons with disabilities and the impact those approaches have on prevalence rates. Their focus is on developing countries.

In another example of a developing country, Helen Namirembe-Nviiri provides information on the various sources of disability data for Uganda and how these data provide information for program design, and resource allocation for persons with disabilities. Her contribution gives a lot of information about the workings of the statistical office in a developing country and the importance of the census in countries without extensive resources for other types of data collection.

Loeb and Eide provide information about other developing African countries, specifically Namibia, Zimbabwe and Malawi. In nationally representative surveys funded by their organization, Sintef, they have applied ICF concepts to the measurement of disability in these locales. The results change the nature of the data available from measures of disability as a state (disabled/not disabled) to a more continuous measure of activity limitations and participation restrictions – giving a more realistic perspective on the experience.

The remaining two papers in that section provide information on the data sources and data collection methods for Brazil and Italy. Chapter 9 provides information about the change in the measures of disability in the Brazilian Decennial Census and the changes in the prevalence that resulted. The expansion of data the new measures provide contribute to a much better understanding of disability in that country, particularly the distribution of labor force participation and the geographic distribution within the country. Crialesi and De Palma approach the data from a different perspective by providing insight into the Italian disability information system and its products. Their discussion demonstrates that in an era of limitations in public resources and the downsizing of welfare programs the efficient organization and use of data on disability becomes an important way of providing necessary information to a diverse audience.

Methodological Issues

The final section of the book hints at the very extensive and broad issues associated with measuring disability in a census or survey context. Ken Black provides a thorough example of the necessity to pre-test census questions and all the subtleties that must be taken into account. Describing the testing process in Australia, Black explains the extensive efforts that the Australian Bureau of Statistics have made to design a measure that will provide a good match between disability identification in the census and in a follow-up survey. The questions raised about false positives and false negatives are important issues to be considered in providing a census question adequate to satisfy the many uses it will have.

Another chapter, written by an Australian, Ros Madden, focuses on the problems of differentiating the ICF components of Activity and Participation when creating questions to be used as measures of those aspects of disability. She identifies a range of measurement issues that need consideration in any ICF measurement application including the need to clarify the purpose before deciding the method, the necessity of understanding the role played by perception in measurement and in addition, the vital role played by people with disabilities in the ICF revision and hopefully in its implementation as well.

Chapter 13 takes another perspective on some of the methodological issues associated with disability measurement. Rasch, Altman and Madans examine the role of assistive devices in the measurement of disability. Accurate measurement is very closely tied to how the respondent interprets the questions and how specific environmental characteristics, such as the use of assistive devices, are included within the questions. The results of their study on data from the National Health Interview Survey indicate that recognition of the impact of the person/environment interaction in developing measures is an important consideration.

The final paper of the volume describes a tool that can be used to focus the methodologist on the issues associated with the multidimensionality of the concept of disability and help in selecting the measure appropriate to the purpose of the data collection. The paper identifies the three major components that need to be considered when trying to reduce the multidimensional model of the ICF to a manageable form for identifying appropriate measures for a survey or census. The authors also provide a guide to understanding the possible purposes for which the data is being collected so that the purpose drives the selection of the domains to be measured rather than using a haphazard collection of questions currently in vogue.

Overall the papers presented here provide some insight into how important disability data is for satisfying the policy needs of the international community, but also how complicated the measurement process has become. Since these papers only reflect the beginnings of the work of the Washington Group, there are many things, such as measuring disability in special populations such as children or among those who are institutionalized that have not been included here. To follow the continued work of the Washington Group please go to the website at http://www.cdc.gov/nchs/citygroup.htm for updates.

REFERENCES

Ingstad, B. (2001). Disability in the developing world. In: G. L. Albrecht, K. D. Seelman & M. Bury (Eds), *Handbook of disability studies* (pp. 772–790). Thousand Oaks, CA: Sage Publications.

Lollar, D. (2001). Public health trends in disability: Past, present and future. In: G. L. Albrecht, K. D. Seelman & M. Bury (Eds), *Handbook of disability studies* (pp. 754–771). Thousand Oaks, CA: Sage Publications.

SECTION I:
BACKGROUND

THE WASHINGTON GROUP: ORIGIN AND PURPOSE

Barbara M. Altman

THE ORIGINS

In June 2001, the United Nations sponsored an international seminar on the measurement of disability. Over a period of three days, a prestigious group of about 90 researchers representing the international community presented papers and discussed the state of measurement of disability in censuses and surveys around the world. The meeting was intended to bring together a broad array of experts in disability measurement from both developed and developing countries in order to evaluate and bring some order to international disability measurement. The focus was to:

1. Review and assess the current status of methods used in population-based data collection activities to measure disability in national statistical systems with particular attention to questionnaire design.
2. Develop recommendations and priorities to advance work on measurement of disability.
3. Contribute to building a network of institutions and experts, including producers and users of disability statistics to implement the developments in this field.
4. Build on accepted international standards and guidelines to achieve these objectives.

International Views on Disability Measures: Moving Toward Comparative Measurement
Research in Social Science and Disability, Volume 4, 9–16

ISSN: 1479-3547/doi:10.1016/S1479-3547(05)04002-9

The participants, who included statisticians from offices in national statistical systems in addition to representatives of the disability community, academic researchers in the field of disability statistics and users of disability data, were provided background documents to facilitate the discussion of the issues. Those documents represented materials from the U.N., the World Health Organization and Eurostat and included the Principles and Recommendations for Population and Housing Censuses, Revision 1, and the International Classification of Functioning, Disabilities and Health (ICF).

In welcoming the prestigious group, Nitin Desai, Under-Secretary General, United Nations Department of Economic and Social Affairs (DESA); Hermann Haberman, Director, United Nations Statistics Division (UNSD); and John Langmore, Director, Division for Social Policy and Development, emphasized the importance of this issue to improving the circumstances of persons with disabilities in the international community and encouraged the efforts of the group.

The early sessions of the meeting provided an historical review of measurement of disability, an overview of instruments used to collect disability data at the national level, with some examination of the adequacy of those instruments, and discussions of the attempts initiated by international organizations for the development of standards and guidelines to measure disability cross-nationally. In the introductory session, Mary Chamie, of the United Nations Statistical Division, presented a very interesting review of the international history of the measurement of disability. She reported that disability statistics are not new. As early as 1950, 33 countries explored the prevalence of disability in their populations without benefit of standardized statistical definitions, concepts or any types of classifications. While this was a start, she asserted that it was not enough to successfully count people. She emphasized that the measurement process must be able to monitor environmental adaptation, the political as well as the cultural environment, and must identify disease and injury patterns.

In that same session, Andre Gubbels, of the European Commission, examined the policy context of the interest in disability data. He made the point that while counting identifies the population, what is done *with* and *for* that population depends on the culture, the policy mandates, and the orientation and interpretation of the data. The disability community's perspective on disability measurement was also shared with the attendees by Yerker Andersson,[1] a member of the National Council on Disability from the U.S. and former president of the World Federation of the Deaf, an international disability organization. Dr. Andersson emphasized the necessity of input of all groups to the measurement process. He was particularly concerned with solely viewing the disablement process from a medical perspective and called for a concerted effort to counteract the view of disability as a medical phenomenon alone. He proposed that the built environment is as much in need of rehabilitation as the individual.

A review of some national experiences in the development of instruments to measure disability provided some interesting discussion. Angela Me and Margaret Mbogoni[2] provided an overview of this process in less-developed countries using data available to them in the UNSD. Of interest was the finding of the variety of definitions of disability that were in use. While a large number of countries adhered to a purely medical definition, in some countries disability was defined in terms of the ability to perform activities. However, few countries defined disability in a social context making reference to participation in domains such as education and work.

Several important themes emerged from this first day including the assessment of the adequacy of and gaps in the instruments in use, the relationship of the instruments to the newly approved ICF, the types of techniques used to harmonize output data and the uses of disability statistics at regional, national and international levels. Overviews of data collected in Europe, which attempted to harmonize conceptualizations and measures, and in less-developed countries provided stark examples of the lack of any standardization of instruments, methodologies or even conceptualization of disability across these different regions of the world. A presentation by Gerry Hendershot[3] during the last session of the day did provide an overview of attempts to address these gaps and provide some coordination of the measurement of disability, particularly in Europe.

The second day of sessions following on an extensive discussion of international initiatives in measurement of disability and statistical techniques from the day before, began with an in-depth discussion of the ICF. Particular attention was paid to the "new" elements associated with the measurement of participation and environment. Presentations highlighted the changes from the ICIDH of 1980 to the ICF approved in 2001. A particular emphasis on the element identified as environment brought this concept, which reflects the physical, social and attitudinal context, into sharp focus and delineated the component parts of that element. The nature of the relationship of the participation element and the environment was highlighted, but the solutions to measurement of these components and their interaction in the census or survey context were not addressed. Another area that received theoretical attention was the differentiation of the activity and participation domains of the ICF, which while separated in the ICF model are currently joined in their presentation in the classification.

Both Ros Madden[4] and Margie Schneider presented papers on the newer elements associated with measurement of disability, participation and environment. Madden's discussion of splitting the Activity and Participation domains is a very useful one for the development of questions that will be used to measure these domains in census or survey formats. Schneider's paper was a very good overview of the participation and environment parts of the ICF, but also contained an interesting and important discussion about a priori definition of disability and a posteriori definition dependent on the structure and orientation of the survey and the variety of questions related to disability included in the survey.

Methodological issues associated with the data collection process and the data collection mechanism also received attention. Difficult issues that arise in collecting data about persons with disabilities including screening questions, use of global questions, question wording and response scales, self/proxy problems were all touched upon. The value of and the problems with using a census for developing the data or health surveys or even special disability surveys were also raised. Experiences from as disparate nations or areas as Australia, Europe and Caribbean countries were reviewed with varied results. The clearest point emerging from the discussion and examples being that no one source of data is workable and foolproof. The discussion of methods and data collection mechanisms highlighted how much work is needed to improve international data on disability.

The last focus of the conference was the additional problems associated with collecting data on special populations, such as children, institutionalized populations and particularly those with cognitive and psychological functioning difficulties. Concurrent working sessions allowed the gathered group of experts to focus on their areas of interest. The reviews of the literature and questions in use combined with examples of activity currently taking place in the field (particularly new childhood measures being used in developing countries) provided a good background on the specialized problems associated with the smaller, but important special populations. While one may have felt overwhelmed by all the information imparted, on the variety of special populations in addition to the conceptual, question language, methodological and data collection mechanism material covered earlier, the results were excellent for establishing the areas where work is still required. The outcome of the intense, three-day meeting was a comprehensive picture of the current state of disability measurement and data collection internationally. The attendees agreed to a person that the meeting provided an excellent starting point to address the issues that had been raised and additionally provided a network of persons interested in doing that work.

In the final session, the rappatour identified eight recommendations coming out of the work that had been done:

- The need for development of principles and standard forms for global indicators to be used in censuses.
- That emphasis be placed on improving the comparability of disability data cross-nationally while being sensitive to the cultural and resource differences encountered among different nations.
- That the ICF be used as the framework for measurement of disability in future work.
- The development of principles for measuring the participation and environment components of the ICF since those are areas of measurement that are still in early stages of elaboration.
- That methodological problems including issues of self vs. proxy respondents, multipoint scale cut points, negative terminology and others be examined depending on interest and time.
- That attention be focused on issues associated with measuring disability among special populations such as children, elderly, institutionalized and others.
- That additional work be done on survey instruments for health surveys and survey supplements that do not focus primarily on disability – as time and interest allow.
- That stakeholders and data users be included in these activities and that exchange of information and establishment of guidelines for the use of data and development of working relationships and networks among countries to further cooperation on disability data topics be stressed.

Following on the discussion of the recommendations by the group, Hermann Habermann, Director of the United Nations Statistical Division called for the creation of a City Group on disability statistics to follow up on the recommendations and work begun at this meeting. He invited the National Center for Health Statistics (NCHS) of the United States to organize the first meeting of the group in Washington, DC within the next year. Based on the tradition associated with City Groups, the group would be known as the Washington Group (WG) based on the location of its first meeting.

ORGANIZATION OF THE WASHINGTON GROUP

The WG on Disability Measurement was formed as a result of the United Nations International Seminar on Measurement of Disability described above. An outcome of that meeting was the recognition that statistical and methodological work was needed at an international level in order to facilitate the comparison of data on disability cross-nationally. Consequently, the United Nations Statistical Division authorized the formation of a City Group to address some of the issues identified in the International Seminar and invited the NCHS, the official health statistics agency of the United States, to host the first meeting of the group. The City Group format is one that has been used by the U.N. in numerous other occasions to address various problems in survey measurement and methodology, such as the Rio Group, which focuses on poverty statistics. The City Group is an informal, temporary organizational format that allows representatives from national statistical agencies to come together to address selected problems in statistical methods. A City Group usually develops a series of three to four working meetings and is named after the location of the first meeting. The first meeting of the WG took place February 18–20, 2002.

THE PURPOSE OF THE WASHINGTON GROUP

As the first order of business, the WG examined the objectives established by the planning committee. At the completion of the sessions and discussions, the group revisited the objectives and refined the wording to better represent the conclusions that had been reached. The following objectives were accepted enthusiastically by the participants and were used to guide the development of a work plan:

1. To guide the development of a small set(s) of general disability measures, suitable for use in censuses, sample-based national surveys, or other statistical formats, which will provide basic necessary information on disability throughout the world.
2. To recommend one or more extended sets of survey items to measure disability or principles for their design, to be used as components of population surveys or as supplements to specialty surveys. These extended sets of survey items will be related to the general measures.
3. Measures identified in objectives 1 and 2 will be culturally comparable to the extent possible. The ICF model, a useful framework to assist in the development of these measures, will be utilized in developing the measures.
4. To address the methodological issues associated with the measurement of disability considered most pressing by the City Group participants.

WASHINGTON GROUP GOVERNANCE

A plan for governance was adopted by the WG at their third meeting in Brussels, February 2004. Representative/s are appointed by the national statistical authorities of member states. Other participants can be included as adjunct members. Adjunct members may participate in the activities of the WG, but they cannot vote in the decision-making process. Adjunct members include well-recognized international organizations with a formal relationship to national statistical authorities such as disability organizations, U.N. affiliates, other statistical agencies (i.e. OECD), organizations that represent national statistical agencies (i.e. Eurostat), and other groups with international expertise in disability statistics.

A key concern of the WG was that there be representation of persons with disabilities. In addition to the European Disability Forum which was already participating at the third meeting, it was agreed that international disability organizations will be identified and invited to participate. This is an ongoing process for the group and continuing efforts are made to include these groups and to provide funding to allow them to attend the meetings.

The NCHS (U.S.A.) was selected as the Executive Secretariat of the WG. A Steering Committee and chair which will be responsible for implementing governance procedures were installed. The Steering Committee will be made up of seven members. These will include three regional members and four hosts of WG Meetings (hosts of three previous meetings and the host for the next upcoming meeting. The Steering Committee is responsible for selecting a Chairperson from among the group of seven. The inaugural Steering Committee was made up of representatives of Canada, Eurostat, the United States, Brazil, Uganda, the Philippines and Egypt. Jennifer Madans of NCHS in the United States was elected as the first Chairperson. The Steering Committee was charged with development of a long-range work plan and timeline for implementation of the work plan to facilitate WG activities.

FURTHER INFORMATION ABOUT THE WASHINGTON GROUP

As this book goes to press, the WG is preparing for its fifth annual meeting to be held in Rio de Janeiro, Brazil in September 2005. The Secretariat maintains a website [at http://www.cdc.gov/nchs/citygroup.htm] which provides ongoing information about the group and their activities. Copies of the presentations made at all the meetings are available as well as any products that the group have produced. Announcements of upcoming meetings with agendas are also placed on the website approximately four months prior to the meeting dates.

NOTES

1. Dr. Andersson's paper is included in this volume, Chapter 5.
2. Dr. Me and Mbogoni's paper, Chapter 6, is included in this volume.
3. Dr. Hendershot's paper is Chapter 3 of this volume.
4. Dr. Madden's paper can be found in this volume, Chapter 12.

SURVEY MEASUREMENT OF DISABILITY: A REVIEW OF INTERNATIONAL ACTIVITIES AND RECOMMENDATIONS

Gerry E. Hendershot

ABSTRACT

Several international and supranational organizations have undertaken efforts to improve and standardize the measurement of disability in population-based surveys. Among these are the Organization for Economic Cooperation and Development, the Statistical Office of the European Commission, the United Nations Statistical Division, the World Health Organization Regional Office for Europe, the World Health Organization, and Réseau sur l'Espérance de Vie en Santé Européennes. In this report their activities and recommendations are reviewed and examined from the viewpoint of the International Classification of Functioning, Disability, and Health.

This paper is excerpted from a more detailed report prepared for the United Nations Statistical Division as a background paper to its International Seminar on the Measurement of Disability, held in New York City,

International Views on Disability Measures: Moving Toward Comparative Measurement
Research in Social Science and Disability, Volume 4, 17–39

ISSN: 1479-3547/doi:10.1016/S1479-3547(05)04003-0

June 4–6, 2001. The report is based on an examination of activities and recommendations of six international and supranational organizations: the Organization for Economic Cooperation and Development (OECD), the Statistical Office of the European Commission (EuroStat), the World Health Organization Regional Office for Europe (EuroWHO), the United Nations Statistical Division (UNSD), the World Health Organization (WHO), and Réseau sur l'Espérance de Vie en Santé Européennes (REVES). Each of these organizations had recently published significant reports on disability measurement in surveys, and those reports were the primary basis for the review. Readers are referred to those reports and the literature they cite for additional details. In this summary of the original report, the activities and recommendations of each of the organizations named above will be briefly reviewed (Part 1), and they will be compared with the World Health Organization's International Classification of Functioning, Disability, and Health (ICF) (Part 2).

PART 1: ACTIVITIES AND RECOMMENDATIONS OF INTERNATIONAL AND SUPRANATIONAL ORGANIZATIONS

Organization for Economic Cooperation and Development

The OECD is an organization of 30 nations who cooperate to create and sustain economic growth in their own countries and in the world. Member states share a commitment to an open market economy, democratic pluralism, and human rights. One of the functions of OECD is to monitor trends in member countries that are related to economic growth and human rights. Because health costs are an important part of the economies of OECD countries, the organization has an active health statistics program. Of particular interest in the field of health is the aging of populations, and resulting changes in health and disability. Disability is also of interest because of OECD's commitment to the human rights of persons with disabilities.

In 1999 an OECD expert meeting on aging and disability observed that policy discussions "are seriously hampered by the lack of internationally comparable data." Whereas many OECD countries had national surveys that included questions on health and disability, there was so little comparability that few international comparisons could be made. In response to that observation, OECD undertook a more careful study of the comparability of national survey data on disability in member countries (Gudex & Lafortune, 2000).

Of the 30 OECD countries, 23 were found to have had a recent national survey that measured health and disability. The questionnaires for each of the surveys were obtained and analyzed with respect to their properties: the definitions of disabilities used, the variety of domains of activity included, etc. Summaries were prepared showing the extent of comparability among surveys with respect to particular properties and in general. Finally, recommendations were made for improving international comparability of disability survey data.

The main contribution of the OECD effort was to identify the broad domains of activity and the specific individual activities within domains that have been used by many surveys in its member countries to identify persons with disabilities. The individual activities for which questions were most comparable across surveys were: the self-care activities of dressing, bathing, and feeding; the mobility activities of climbing, walking, and transferring (from bed to chair), and the communication activities of seeing, hearing, and speaking. The fact that many countries operationally define disability using these domains and activities suggests that they are useful and feasible measures to include in other surveys.

The existence of a degree of consensus on survey measures of disability within OECD countries should not obscure another key finding of the OECD inventory: even among this group of countries that is relatively homogeneous with respect to economic development, the degree of comparability among most survey measures of disability remains low.

Statistical Office of the European Commission

Through its Task Force on Health and Health-related Survey Data, the Statistical Office of the European Commission (Eurostat) supported a Danish National Institute of Public Health (NIPH) survey of disability data collected in the European Union (EU) (Gudex, Christensen, & Rasmussen, 1999). The survey covered 16 national surveys by 11 EU member states. Questions from each survey were classified by general topic in the following categories: chronic problems, acute problems, limited daily activities, physical and sensory functioning, work participation, occupational status, educational level, and employment status.[1] The questions in each category were compared across surveys with respect to format, wording, and meaning, and judgments were made about the comparability of questions and categories across countries. It was concluded that,

> Overall, comparability is low between surveys and there are no surveys which could be compared on all or most questions. For most of the disability-related indicators, however, there are some comparisons which may be useful, where there are approximately 6–8 surveys asking a similar question (Gudex et al., 1999, p. 40).

The activity domains for which this criterion was met (similar questions in 6 or more surveys) were climbing stairs (7 surveys), running or walking (6 surveys), lying down and getting up (6), bending forward or kneeling (6), being confined to one's home (6), using the toilet (6), dressing or undressing (6), having speaking difficulties (6), and feeding one's self (6).

World Health Organization Regional Office for Europe

In the late 1980s and early 1990s, the World Health Organization Regional Office for Europe (EuroWHO) and Statistics Netherlands undertook a series of consultations with representatives of European national health interview surveys. The project went under the name EUROHIS, for European Health Interview Surveys. The goal of EUROHIS was to harmonize European health interview survey measures of health targets in WHO's "Health for All" program. (The word "harmonize" is often used in international, especially European, discussions of classifications from different nations, and means to bring into agreement.) Three consultations were held (1988, 1990, and 1992), leading to the publication of "Health Interview Surveys: Toward international harmonization of methods and instruments" (deBruin & Picavet, 1996).

In the area of long-term disability, EUROHIS explicitly adopted the framework of the International Classification of Impairments, Disabilities, and Handicaps (World Health Organization, 1980), or ICIDH, and even provided ICIDH code values for the disability questions it recommended. The activity domains for which questions were recommended were: walking, transferring (in and out of bed and chair), dressing, bathing, feeding one's self, using the toilet, hearing, and seeing. EUROHIS has also tested an 8-item quality of life instrument that includes a disability related item: "satisfaction with ability to perform daily living activities." In November 2000 EUROHIS held a mid-term review of its work (EUROHIS, 2000). Twenty-seven European countries, the OECD, and WHO were represented.

At that point, common instruments had been developed and tested for most topics, including disability.

World Health Organization

The World Health Organization Disability Assessment Schedule II (WHODAS II) has been developed by the Assessment, Classification, and Epidemiology group (ACE), a unit in the Global Programe on Evidence for Health Policy (GPE) at the World Health Organization headquarters in Geneva, Switzerland. The ACE group is also responsible for the International Classification of Impairments, Disabilities, and Health (World Health Organization, 2001) or ICF, and the International Classification of Diseases (World Health Organization, 1992) or (ICD).

The direct antecedent of WHODAS II was the World Health Organization Psychiatric Disability Schedule (WHO/DAS) published in 1988. WHO/DAS was used to assess disability in psychiatric patients in a number of dimensions of behavior. WHODAS II is a complete revision of WHO/DAS. It was undertaken with several objectives in mind. First, it was intended to be compatible with the revised ICIDH, now the ICF. Second, it was intended to be cross-culturally applicable; that is, it was intended to be useful in places that differ in language, history, and custom. Third, WHODAS II was intended to treat all disorders at parity; that is, it was intended to be useful when evaluating disabilities of all kinds: mental, physical, sensory, and so on. This objective was based on the assumption that functioning is an important measure of outcomes, regardless of its determinants.

WHODAS II assesses functioning in six domains: understanding and communicating, getting around, self care, getting along with others, household and work activities, and participation in society. In each domain 4–6 questions are asked about the person's difficulty in doing specific behaviors; for instance, in the domain of self-care, questions are asked about washing and eating. For each reported behavior difficulty information is obtained on the frequency of that difficulty by asking on how many days (in the last 30 days) the difficulty occurred.

WHODAS II is available in several versions. WHO recommends that its 36-item version be used, administered by an interviewer in a face-to-face interview with the person whose function is being assessed. If that is not possible, WHO offers 36-item versions for self-administration by the subject and for self-administration by a proxy for the subject. There is also a

36-item version for administration by an interviewer to a proxy respondent. For circumstances in which 36 items are too numerous, there are 12-item versions for interviewer – and self-administration, and 6-item versions for administration by proxies and clinicians.

In its annual report for the year 2000, The World Health Report 2000, the World Health Organization presented a system for measuring the performance of national health systems (World Health Organization, 2000a). According to the report, five things must be measured to assess a population's health system: level of health, equality of health, level of responsiveness, equality of responsiveness, and equality of financing. Each of these measurements are at the population level; that is, for instance, "level of health" refers to an assessment of the health of the population as a whole, which may be estimated by aggregating health measures for individual persons. For each of these five aspects of a health system, methods were proposed for calculating a numerical score, and scores were calculated for WHO member states. The scores for the five aspects were combined in a weighted overall score for each national health system.

The aspect of the WHO assessment system relevant to this review is health. One-half of the overall score comprises "level of health" (25%) and "equality of health" (25%). "Health" is measured by Disability Adjusted Life Expectancy (DALE), a summary measure of population health. The level of health for a health system is the DALE for the population it serves, and the equality of health is a statistic measuring the evenness of distribution of DALE across socioeconomic subgroups of that population. The method for computing DALE is presented in the report from WHO (2000a). (The WHO report, especially its method for measuring population health, was the cause of considerable controversy: for one critical view, see Navarro, 2001.)

Like other summary measures of population health, to calculate a DALE requires data on population mortality and morbidity. Whereas comparable data on mortality are available for many nations, internationally comparable data on morbidity (nonfatal health outcomes) are scarce. The WHO staff noted that "First, no single instrument (for measuring morbidity) appears to be commonly used internationally," and "Second…no instrument has proven cross-population comparability" (World Health Organization, September, 2000b). It was recommended, therefore, that the "WHO Secretariat should orchestrate the development and periodic implementation of a common survey instrument for measuring health states."

According to WHO, the most important problem in international comparability is a lack of "cross-national comparability." That is, different populations have different expectations about health, and therefore respond differently to questions that may otherwise be reliable, valid, cross-culturally applicable, and intra-culturally consistent. For instance, a response that is scored as "excellent health" in one population often does not correspond to the same true general health condition as a response that is scored as "excellent health" in another population (Sadana, Mathers, Lopez, Murray, & Iburg, 2000).

WHO proposes three approaches to achieving cross-population comparability. First, compare survey measures with authoritative objective measures ("calibration tests"); for instance, compare survey reports of seeing limitations with standard clinical tests of vision for the same persons. Second, use coding rules for survey measures to code standardized descriptions of the health of individual persons ("standard case vignettes"). Third, administer the survey instrument to populations whose health is known to be very good ("reference cases").

The health and health-related domains to be included in surveys by WHO are selected from the ICF, as follows: Vision, hearing, speech, digestion, bodily excretion, fertility, sexual activity, skin/disfigurement, breathing, pain, affect, sleep, energy/vitality, cognition, communication, mobility, dexterity, self-care, usual activities, social functioning, and interpersonal relations. Questions for these domains have been developed and tested and are now used in WHO-sponsored national health surveys in many nations. Many of the questions are identical to, or variations of, questions in WHODAS II.

Réseau sur l'Espérance de Vie en Santé Européennes

REVES (in English, "International Network on Health Expectancy and the Disability Process") is an international association of researchers who share an interest in "health expectancy." EuroREVES is a subgroup of REVES comprising European scientists. Health expectancy combines mortality and morbidity data to estimate the number of healthy years of life that can be expected by a cohort of newborns in a particular population, given current rates of mortality and morbidity. The DALE measure used by WHO (mentioned in the preceding section) is one approach to measuring life expectancy.

With support from the Health Monitoring Program of the Commission of European Communities (EC), EuroREVES undertook to review international recommendations and practices in survey measurement of health, and to propose standard measures for use by surveys in European Union. They reported the results in Selection of a Coherent Set of Health Indicators: A First Step Toward a User's Guide to Health Expectancies for the European Union (Robine, Jagger, & Egedi, 2000). As the title suggests, the project was undertaken with the long-run goal of standardizing measures of health and increasing the comparability of health expectancies.

The study focuses on five aspects of health: physical and sensory limitations, activity restrictions in daily life, limitations in usual activities, perceived health, and mental health. The first three of these domains are relevant to this paper. The domains proposed for physical and sensory abilities are shown in Box 1. The domains proposed for activities of daily living are feeding, transferring, dressing, bathing, and toileting. Although question wording had not been completely worked out at the time of the report, the general approach was to ask about abilities with and without the assistance of other persons or special equipment.

EuroREVES proposed that a single question be asked about "usual activities," which could then be used as a summary measure or "global indicator" of disability (Verbrugge, Merrill, & Liu, 1999). The wording proposed for that question is shown in Box 2. A global indicator is useful for describing disability, explaining disability, and screening for disability. It is

Box 1. Physical and Sensory Abilities Proposed by Euro-REVES.

Seeing newspaper print	Seeing a face at 4 meters
Hearing another person	Keeping balance
Walking 500 meters	Climbing 12 stairs

Box 2. Global Indicator.

"For the past 6 months or more have you been limited in activities people usually do because of a health problem?"

Yes, strongly limited/Yes, limited/No, not limited

useful for describing disability because an indicator based on one or a few questions is inherently easier to understand and communicate than an indicator based on many questions. It is useful for explaining disability because it can be used as a predictor or an outcome variable in causal models, and it can be transported across a variety of research settings and disciplines, adding to the scope of information that can be related to disability. It is useful in screening for disability in situations in which it is desirable to first determine efficiently if a person has a disability before asking a series of additional questions about the disability or its consequences.

United Nations Statistical Division

In 1993 the General Assembly of the United Nations adopted the Standard Rules for the Equalization of Opportunity for Persons with Disabilities (hereinafter, "the Rules"; United Nations, 1994). Its purpose is "to ensure that girls, boys, women and men with disabilities, as members of their societies, may exercise the same rights and obligations as others" (paragraph 15).

For several reasons the Rules are important for statistical measurement of disability. First, they adopt a set of "fundamental concepts" that provide parameters for operationally defining disability. Second, they identify the program and policy areas for which measurement is needed. And third, they establish guidelines for data systems to measure disability.

In identifying fundamental concepts of disability, the Rules make distinctions between several levels or dimensions of "disability." While they use ICIDH nomenclature, the discussion is consistent with the ICF concepts of "activity limitation," "participation restriction," and "environmental barrier." There was an explicit attempt to conceptualize disability in a way that would be useful for preventing disability, rehabilitating persons with disability, and equalizing opportunities for persons with disabilities. The resulting conceptualization of disability was meant for broad application in medical care, rehabilitation services, and human rights.

In addition to identifying fundamental concepts and policy-relevant areas of social life, the Rules make specific recommendations for disability data systems. The recommendations, although brief, are very comprehensive. They call for disability data from censuses and surveys, for data on many different aspects of disability, and for data at geographic levels from national to local. They call for setting standards for nomenclature and methods of data collection, and for the widespread sharing of findings and field experience. One rule calls for the full participation of persons with disabilities in all aspects of disability data systems, as survey planners, data collectors, study subjects, and research analysts.

As part of its efforts to foster greater international comparability of disability data, in compliance with the Rules, the UNSD prepared a new section of the UN's Principles and Recommendations for Population and Housing Censuses, Revision 1 (United Nations, 1998). The authors made several key recommendations for collecting disability information in national censuses. While commending the ICIDH as a conceptual framework, the authors noted that the Impairment and Handicap dimensions of the ICIDH (now Impairment and Participation Restriction in the International Classification of Functioning (ICF) are difficult to measure in censuses. They recommended, instead, that Disability (Activity Limitation in the ICF) be measured, because it can be done with relatively few and simple questions. Further, to fit disability questions into brief census schedules, the authors recommend that a short list of disabilities be measured (Box 3).

The Statistical Division has produced two other, more detailed documents on disability statistics: a Manual for the Development of Statistical Information for Disability Programes and Policies (United Nations, 1996), and Guidelines and Principles for the Development of Disability Statistics (United Nations, 2001). The Manual is addressed to policy staff

Box 3. Disability Types for Which The United Nations Statistical Division Recommends Collecting Census Data.

Seeing difficulties (even with glasses, if worn)
Hearing difficulties (even with eyeglasses, if worn)
Speaking difficulties (talking)
Moving/Mobility (walking, climbing stairs, standing)
Body movement difficulties (reaching, crouching, kneeling)
Gripping/holding difficulties (using fingers to grasp or handle objects)
Learning difficulties (intellectual difficulties, retardation)
Behavioral difficulties (psychological, emotional problems)
Personal care difficulties (bathing, dressing, feeding)
Others

members who are not statisticians, whereas the Guidelines are addressed to statisticians. Both documents recommend using the ICF as the conceptual model for collecting and presenting disability data.

PART 2: COMPARISON TO THE INTERNATIONAL CLASSIFICATION OF FUNCTIONING, DISABILITY AND HEALTH

In this section comparisons are made between the International Classification of Functioning Disability and Health (ICF) (World Health Organization, 2001) and the recommendations made by the six international and supranational organizations whose recent reports have been reviewed: the OECD, the EuroStat, the EuroWHO, the WHO, REVES, and the UNSD. The comparisons are organized around some key conceptual and operational issues in the ICF.

The Distinction between Activity and Participation

The ICF makes a distinction between "activity" and "participation." At the beginning of the revision process these were originally conceptualized as "dimensions" or "levels" of disability, corresponding in a general sense to the "disability" and "handicap" dimensions of ICIDH 1980. Activity was conceived to refer to the person level of disability and participation to the social or societal level. Further, it was conceived that within each dimension there were plural "domains," broad categories of personal activities and societal participation, and that within those broad categories were many specific activities and types of participation that comprised the detailed categories of the classification system.

Toward the end of the revision process, however, it became clear that a consensus could not be achieved on which domains should be included in Activity and which should be included in Participation. The lack of consensus resulted from disagreement about the definitions of personal and social: what was clearly "personal activity" to one participant was just as clearly "social participation" to another participant, and vice versa.

Eventually WHO decided that all domains were both personal and social and that users could code them as Activity, or Participation, or both Activity and Participation. One list of domains and detailed categories within domains was to be used which ever, Activity or Participation, was being coded. The same code number was to be assigned to a detailed category whether it was coded as Activity, or Participation, or both. A literal prefix would indicate which was being coded, "a" for Activity and "p" for Participation; or if the user chose not to make the distinction between A and P, the generic prefix "d" (for disability) could be substituted. Thus, for instance, in a study of housing and disability, "acquiring a place to live" could be assigned ICF code **a**610 if the focus were on the person level (reading newspaper advertisements, talking to realtors, etc.) or **p**610 if the focus were on the societal level (discriminatory housing practices, business cycles, etc.) Or if the emphasis were on both or neither, it could be coded **d**610.

Given the history of this issue in the ICIDH revision, it is interesting to examine how it is handled in the recommendations of international and supranational organizations. The EUROHIS recommendation on disability adopted the ICIDH 1980 framework of three "planes of experience" in the consequences of disease: impairments, disabilities, and handicaps, which correspond, respectively, to effects on the body, the person, and the society. Therefore, the questions recommended by EUROHIS are labeled as pertaining to Handicap (3 questions on mobility) or Disability (10 questions on self-care, continence, hearing, and seeing).

The EuroREVES document also distinguishes between levels of disability, using a scheme first presented by Philip Wood (1975). The pertinent levels of the scheme for EuroREVES are "functional limitations" and "activity restriction." Functional limitation is conceived by EuroREVES to be a person-level dimension, whereas activity restriction is conceived to be at the social level. While activity limitation might encompass different social roles, EuroREVES focuses on independent self-care, measured with questions about feeding, transferring, dressing, toileting, and bathing. The distinction between functional limitations and activity restriction is said by EuroREVES to be important for policy purposes because the choice of a preventive intervention may be conditioned by the causal relationship between the two levels of disability.

The documents of the UN Statistical Division that were reviewed recommended an approach to disability that makes clear distinctions between dimensions of disability pertaining to body, person, and community. Indeed, it argues that such distinctions are necessary to implement programs and policies consistent with the Standard Rules. Because the documents were prepared early in the ICIDH revision process, they reflect the view prevailing at that time that the revised classification would preserve such distinctions.

WHODAS II was developed and began testing during a phase of the ICIDH revision in which a distinction was still being made between Activity and Participation as being at the person and societal levels, respectively. WHODAS II assesses disability in six "domains," which include what were, at the time of its development, Activities and Participation domains. The structure of the questions is the same across all of the domains measured, and they have been shown to be empirically distinct. The domains are treated, in effect, as undifferentiated with respect the levels they represent, anticipating the ultimate WHO position on the ICF: with respect to their content, there is no necessary distinction between Activity domains and Participation domains.

In summary, the position now taken by WHO in the ICF and WHODAS-II is apparently at odds with the positions taken by EUROHIS, EuroREVES, and UNSD. The latter regard a distinction between the person and social levels as being scientifically correct and practically useful, whereas the former regards the distinction as unnecessary, potentially confusing, and therefore optional.

The Distinction between Performance and Capacity

Another late innovation to the ICF was the distinction between "performance" and "capacity." During most of the revision process, the emphasis had been placed on what people can be observed to do, whether as individuals (activity) or as participants in social life (participation). A complication of this approach was recognized: what a person does may depend on their use or nonuse of personal assistance and special equipment. To address this complication, it was proposed that the coding scheme allow for noting whether the assessment was made with or without personal assistance or special equipment.

The ultimate ICF retained that feature and added a new feature that allows for assessing function in the person's actual environment, called "Performance," and in a standardized environment, called "Capacity." Combining the two environmental conditions (actual and standardized) and the two assistance conditions (with and without personal or technological help), there are four sets of conditions for assessing function.

In the coding scheme, a specific digital position is reserved for each set of assessment conditions, following the three-digit domain code and a decimal-point divider (Box 4). The numeric entry in each place indicates the extent of difficulty in performing the activity or participation under the specified

Box 4. ICF Code Structure for Activity or Participation.

Activity or Participation ↓		Does do (with help) in current environment ↓	Could do without help in standard environment ↓	Could do with help in standard environment ↓	Does do without help in current Environment ↓
___ ___ ___	●	______	______	______	______
3 digit domain code	↑ Decimal-point separator	1st qualifier	2nd qualifier	3rd qualifier	4th qualifier

Qualifier values (amount of difficulty under specified conditions):
0 = NONE, 1 = MILD, 2 = MODERATE, 3 = SEVERE,
4 = COMPLETE

conditions of environment and assistance, with values from 0 (no difficulty) to 4 (complete difficulty).

The ICF coding scheme for activity and participation allows a rich body of information to be recorded in a simple and direct manner. To take full advantage of the coding scheme, however, requires that a large amount of information be collected: information about Activity or Participation in sufficient detail to assign ICF domain codes, information about the use of personal assistance and assistive technology, and assessments of five levels of difficulty in both a current environment and a standardized environment.

None of the question sets currently recommended by international organizations would provide all of this information. Table 1 shows the ICF information requirements – two environmental conditions (columns 2 and 3) and two assistance conditions (columns 4 and 5), the four qualifiers constructed from those conditions (columns 6–9), and the five levels of severity to be assessed (cell entries in columns 6–9). Below the ICF row are rows for each of the major internationally recommended disability questionnaires. Cell entries indicate whether or not the ICF-required information is available from the recommended questions (columns 2–5), and the levels of severity available (columns 6–9).

All of the recommended questionnaires ask about performance in the current environment (column 3), making it possible for them to assess qualifier 1 (column 6). Also, all of the recommended question sets could assess qualifier 1 at several levels of severity of limitation or participation, although only WHODAS 2 has all five levels recommended by the ICF.

There is some ambiguity, however, in the EUROHIS questions with respect to the environmental condition required for qualifiers 1 and 2. The preamble to the questions specifies that they refer "to what you are normally capable of doing," and the questions about specific activities begin "Can you ...." The words "capable" and "can", may connote in English an implied "standardized environment" that is different from the actual current environment. That is, a person could interpret the question to mean "given the best circumstances, how difficult is it for you to ...?" rather than "given your actual circumstances, how difficult is it for you to ...?" If the former is understood, a kind of "standardized" favorable environment is implied, but it is not clearly specified.

The ambiguity in the EUROHIS questions in this regard points to the subtlety in distinctions between performance in actual environments and capacity in standard environments. Questions must be formulated that distinguish between what a person "does do" (performance) and what a person "can do" (capacity). It has yet to be tested whether or not survey respondents can make these distinctions reliably and validly.

Table 1. ICF Activity and Participation Codes Compared to Recommended Survey Questions.

Measurement Recommendation	Performance (current environment)	Capacity (standard environment)	Without Assistance (person or equipment)	With Assistance (person or equipment)	Does do (with help, if needed) in Current Environment	Could do Without Help in Standard Environment	Could do with Help in Standard Environment	Does do Without Help in Current Environment
(1)	(2)	(3)	(4)	(5)	(6)	(7)	(8)	(9)
ICF	Yes	Yes	Yes	Yes	No Mild Moderate Severe Complete	No Mild Moderate Severe Complete	No Mild Moderate Severe Complete	No Mild Moderate Severe Complete
EUROHIS	Yes	No	Yes	Yes (personal assistance only)	None Lower Higher Unable	No	No	None Lower Unable
EuroREVES	Yes	No	Yes	Yes	None Light Moderate Severe	No	No	Yes
WHODAS II	Yes	No	No	No	None Mild Moderate Severe Extreme/can not do	No	No	No

None of the recommended questionnaires inquires about performance in standardized environments (column 3), with the possible exception of EUROHIS, as just noted. Therefore, none is able to assess qualifiers 2 and 3 (columns 7 and 8). Also, because WHODAS II does not ask explicitly about performance without assistance, it cannot assess qualifier 4 (column 8). The EUROHIS and EuroREVES recommended questions would support assessment of qualifier 4, because both ask explicitly about performance with and without assistance.

Selecting Domains of Activity and Participation

Much of the work by international and supranational organizations reviewed in this report was concerned with the domains and subdomains of human life that should be included in survey measurements of disability. It was apparent in the review of that work that some areas of broad consensus already exist. In this section the areas of consensus will be identified within the framework of the ICF, which will also identify the areas of the ICF framework most in need of further development.

Table 2 shows in the left column the chapter numbers and titles of the Activity and Participation dimensions of the ICF. Each of the remaining columns of Table 2 refers to an organization whose recent reports were reviewed earlier in this paper. In the case of WHO, two activities are shown separately: the WHODAS II activity and the health system assessment activity. In the case of UNSD, the findings of several of its recent documents are collapsed into a single column.

An X in a cell of Table 2 indicates the author's judgment that the organization in that column has "recommended" that the ICF domain identified in the first column be included in survey measurements of disability. Recommended is in quotation marks because some organizations did not so much recommend the use of a domain as observe its frequent use among the surveys it reviewed. This amounts to assuming that a widely used domain is recommended for use. While all nine chapters of the Activity and Participation dimensions are shown in the first column, only the subdomains in which recommendations were made are listed.

With regard to the domains recommended by the international and supranational organizations, few correspond to the domains in ICF chapters 1, 2, 6, and 9 (highlighted in Table 2). If survey measures are to cover the full range of ICF domains, these are obviously areas in which developmental work is needed. On the other hand, ICF Chapters 3, 4, 5, 7,

Table 2. Coverage of ICF Activity and Participation Domains by Survey Questionnaire Items Recommended or Most Commonly Used, According to Source.

ICF Activity and Participation Domains	OECD	EuroStat	EUROHIS	WHODAS	WHO Quex	Euro REVES	UNSD
1. Learning and applying knowledge					X		X
2. General tasks and demands							
3. Communication							
Receiving spoken messages (hearing)	X	X	X		X	X	X
Receiving nonverbal messages (seeing)	X	X	X		X	X	X
Speaking	X	X	X	X	X	X	X
4. Mobility							
Changing and maintaining body position	X	X	X	X		X	X
Carrying, moving, and handling objects				X	X	X	X
Walking and moving	X	X	X	X		X	X
5. Self-care							
Washing		X	X	X		X	X
Eating	X	X		X		X	X
Toileting		X	X			X	
Dressing		X	X	X			X
6. Domestic life				X			
7. Interpersonal interactions and relationships				X	X	X	X
8. Major life areas	X	X	X	X	X	X	X
9. Community, social and civic life				X			

and 8 more frequently had matches to recommended questions, which is not to say that all subdomains in those chapters would be measured if the recommendations were all adopted; on the contrary, many subdomains in those chapters are not listed in Table 2 because no organization recommended items corresponding to those domains.

With regard to ICF Chapter 2, in which no recommendations are listed, a further comment is in order. The ICF says in the introduction to activity and participation Chapter 2, "General tasks and demands":

> This chapter is about general aspects of carrying out single or multiple tasks, organizing routines, and handling stress. These items can be used with more specific tasks or actions to identify the underlying features of the execution of tasks under different circumstances (World Health Organization, 2001, p. 129).

This is a new concept not present in the ICIDH and not present in the thinking of the organizations whose work has been reviewed here. Clearly on the basis of the evidence reviewed in this report, this is a domain in which additional research is needed.

Further comment also is in order concerning ICF Activity and Participation Chapter 8 on major life areas, about which the ICF says:

> This chapter is about engaging in and carrying out the tasks and actions required to perform education, work and employment, and economic transactions (World Health Organization, 2001, p. 164).

All organizations are credited with having "recommended" measures in this area, but this could be misleading. Several of the organizations do recommend questions specially designed to measure limitations in work activity or usual activity (which would include work or school in most societies). Others, however, do not recommend specific measures of work disability, but do recommend or assume that usual activities such as work, education, and economic activities will be collected as "demographic variables" in any survey on disability, and that such measures will be used to measure the relative participation of persons with and without disability. UNSD, for instance, includes work activity as one of the outcome variables to tabulate according to various measures of activity limitation.

The conventional inclusion on some surveys of questions that can be used to measure participation in major life activities is fortunate. However, in the future, measuring participation in major life activities should be more formally and explicitly related to the concept as formulated in the ICF. The conventional range of major life activities in surveys, often including play, school, work, and home management, should be broadened. Furthermore, those measures should be made both for persons with disabilities and those without, so that comparisons of participation rates can be made.

The ICF Activity and Participation Chapter 9 on community, social, and civic life is a major step in that direction. Its subdomains include community life (formal and informal associations, and ceremonies), recreation and leisure (play, sports, art and culture, crafts, hobbies, and socializing), religion and spirituality, human rights, and citizenship. If measures were taken of the participation in all of those major life activities, for persons with and without disabilities, much more would be known about the gaps in participation caused by activity, limitations, and environmental barriers.

Long Forms, Short Forms, and Global Indicators

A good case has been made by EuroREVES and WHO that short forms of questionnaires on functioning are needed for a variety of purposes. Most importantly, perhaps, functioning is a very general aspect of human life, and is therefore relevant to many fields of study. It is therefore desirable to include measures of functioning in data sets covering a wide range of human experiences, such as labor force participation, medical encounters, criminal victimization, etc.

However, specialists in each of these broad fields of human experience have their own data needs, and given typical limitations on resources (including respondent burden), they cannot collect a lot of data on functioning. The only realistic hope for obtaining functional information in these diverse fields is to reduce the amount of such information to a minimum, perhaps even to a single question.

This need has been recognized by EuroREVES and by WHODAS II. EuroREVES recommends a Global Indicator of Activity Limitation (GALI), and WHODAS II offers a 12-item short form of its recommended 36-item questionnaire. EUROHIS does not currently offer a short form, although it should be noted that its full set of recommended questions is not very long to begin with.

While these efforts are worthwhile and should be continued, there is a need to link them more closely to the ICF. In terms of ICF concepts, domains, and categories, what are these short form questionnaire and global indicators measuring? Do they measure impairments, activity limitations, participation restrictions, or something else?

Measures of Environmental Factors

One of the major improvements in the ICF over its predecessor is the recognition of "external factors," primarily the physical and social environment, as major determinants of all three dimensions of functioning and disability, especially of participation. In the reports reviewed here, the environment was occasionally mentioned, but nowhere were specific recommendations made concerning its measurement. Indeed, the inclusion of environment is so new to surveys on disability, that hardly any thought has been given to how to measure it in a survey situation. This is perhaps the largest single gap between the current state of disability survey methodology and the data requirements of the ICF. It is not necessary to delay progress on other fronts to close this gap, but neither is there any excuse for not beginning immediately to develop and implement workable survey measures of environmental barriers and facilitators.

Including Persons with Disabilities in Survey Processes

Of the documents reviewed for this report, only the United Nations documents emphasized the importance of including persons with disabilities in the processes of designing, implementing, and disseminating disability surveys and in the process of being a survey respondent. That does not mean, of course, that the organizations that produced the other documents do not agree with the UN on this point – they most assuredly do. In its revision of the ICIDH, for instance, WHO actively sought and frequently heeded the advice persons of persons with disabilities and of the organizations representing them. What is missing, however, even in the UN manual for disability program managers and the UN guidelines for survey researchers, is practical guidance on methods for involving persons with disabilities in the survey process as survey designers, survey researchers, and survey respondents.

This paper has documented a wide array of activities by international and supranational organizations in the field of disability measurement in surveys and censuses that were occurring near the end of the 20th century. Those activities have continued and expanded in the early 21st century; for instance, as a result of the international conference for which this paper was first prepared, the United Nations Statistical Division has inaugurated an international study of disability measurement in surveys and censuses, which at this writing has met four times, in Washington, DC (which gave the activity its name, "The Washington City Group"); Ottawa, Canada; Brussels, Belgium; and Bangkok, Thailand. Fortunately, the scientists and policy analysts involved in these measurement activities share commitments to collaboration and cooperation in their efforts to improve disability statistics around the world. As their efforts continue to bear fruit, we can expect that there will be a better evidence base for national and international policy on disability. Better policies will help to achieve the United Nations' goal: insuring that "that girls, boys, women and men with disabilities, as members of their societies, may exercise the same rights and obligations as others."

NOTES

1. The terminology of the original report has been retained in this list, as it has, generally, in the brief reviews of other reports included herein.

REFERENCES

deBruin, A., & Picavet, H. S. J. (1996). *Health interview surveys: Towards international harmonization of methods and instruments*. Copenhagen and Voorgurg: WHO Regional Series, European Series, No. 58.

EUROHIS. (2000). *Common methods and instruments for health interview surveys in Europe*. Report of the EUROHIS mid-term review. Copenhagen, November 2–4.

Gudex, C., Christensen, S. H., & Rasmussen, N. (1999). *Survey data on disability*. Eurostat working papers, Population and social conditions, No. 20. Luxembourg: European Commision.

Gudex, C., & Lafortune, G. (2000). *An inventory of health and disability-related surveys in OECD countries*. Labour Market and Social Policy-Occasional Papers No. 44. Paris: OECD.

Navarro, V. (2001). The new conventional wisdom: An evaluation of the WHO report, health systems: Improving performance. *International Journal of Health Services*, *31*(1), 23–33.

Robine, J. M., Jagger, C., & Egedi, V. (2000). *Selection of a coherent set of health indicators*. Montpellier (France): Euro-REVES.

Sadana, R., Mathers, C. D., Lopez, A., Murray, C. J. L., & Iburg, K. (2000). *Comparative analyses of more than 50 household surveys on health status*. GPE Discussion Paper Series: No. 15. Geneva: World Health Organization.

United Nations. (1994). *Standard rules for the equalization of opportunity for persons with disabilities*. New York: United Nations.

United Nations. (1996). *Manual for the development of statistical information for disability programs and policies. Statistics on special population groups* (Series Y, No. 8). New York: United Nations.

United Nations. (1998). *Principles and recommendations for population and housing censuses*, Revision 1. Statistical papers, Series M, No. 67/Rev. 1. New York: United Nations.

United Nations. (2001). *Guidelines and principles for the development of disability statistics (Draft)*. New York: United Nations.

Verbrugge, L. M., Merrill, S. S., & Liu, X. (1999). Measuring disability with parsimony. *Disability and Rehabilitation*, *21*(5/6), 295–306.

World Health Organization. (1980). *International classification of impairments, disabilities, and handicaps*. Geneva: World Health Organization.

World Health Organization. (1992). *International statistical classification of diseases and related health problems (tenth revision)*. Geneva: World Health Organization.

World Health Organization. (2000a). *The world health report, 2000 – health systems: Improving performance*. Geneva: World Health Organization.

World Health Organization. (2000b). *Measuring and reporting of the health of populations*. Background document for the Executive Board resolution on reporting on health of the populations. Geneva: World Health Organization.

World Health Organization. (2001). *International classification of functioning, disability, and health*. Geneva: World Health Organization.

CULTURAL BELIEFS AND PRACTICES THAT INFLUENCE THE TYPE AND NATURE OF DATA COLLECTED ON INDIVIDUALS WITH DISABILITY THROUGH NATIONAL CENSUS

Nora Groce

ABSTRACT

Collection of data about disability in a census or survey context is influenced by the cultural context, particularly the beliefs and practices within the communities where the data are collected. Attitudes toward individuals with disability will influence what questions are asked, how such questions are framed, and how individuals in the community will respond to these questions. This article examines how culturally defined concepts of disability influence the development of questions on the topic, as well as helps determine who asks the questions and who answers the questions. These issues in turn influence how much data are collected and how accurate the data are. It also examines how ethnic diversity and poverty contribute to these questions. Recommendations for attention to these issues are made by census and survey.

International Views on Disability Measures: Moving Toward Comparative Measurement
Research in Social Science and Disability, Volume 4, 41–54

ISSN: 1479-3547/doi:10.1016/S1479-3547(05)04004-2

INTRODUCTION

One of the major impediments to improving services for and advocacy on behalf of disabled populations is the lack of accurate and comparable bodies of epidemiological and demographic data. Until a solid understanding of the size and diversity of the disabled population within a nation is known, politicians, ministers of finance, health and education, and heads of international development organizations will be able to continue to ignore many of the most pressing needs and concerns of the disability community. Numbers *are* strength. However, accurate numbers are necessary – both to be able to demand the political attention that is warranted – and just as importantly – to be able to meet the actual needs of those who live with a disability. Resources will always be finite – the need to know what local, regional, and national disabled populations look like and how they rank their own needs is therefore imperative.

BACKGROUND

Although collection of census information is approached as though it were largely free of social and cultural constraints, in fact, it is important to acknowledge that responses to all censuses have the potential to be influenced by the beliefs and practices of the communities in which the data is collected. This is nowhere more true than in the collection of data regarding individuals with a disability and disabled populations.

Attitudes toward individuals with disability will influence what questions are asked, how such questions are framed, and how individuals in the community will respond to these questions. In many cases, cultural beliefs will also play a role in how census takers themselves approach (or avoid) collection of certain types of data.

Collection of accurate data on disability in many countries is problematic. It is a "Catch 22" situation: to improve social integration and to address social and economic needs of individuals with disability, policy makers need data. However, census collection of data about disability can be hampered by the very social stigmas associated with disability for which the data are needed if changes are to be made.

There are a number of ways of conceptualizing the limitations to data collection that might be imposed by cultural and social attitudes toward disability. In this particular paper, three of the most prominent issues will be addressed.

1. Culturally defined concepts of disability which may limit the types of questions being asked in census collection.
2. Limitations imposed by who is asking the questions (i.e. cultural constraints faced by census takers).
3. Limitations imposed by who is answering the questions (cultural constraints faced by household informants).

The title of the session at the Washington City Group meeting for which this paper was initially prepared was "Unique Cultural Practices that Influence the Nature of the Environment or Prescribe or Proscribe Participation." An attempt will be made here to cover both prescriptions and proscriptions that might be involved, however, the idea of enumerating "unique" cultural practices has been reframed. This is because responses to disability cross-culturally often fall into recognizable patterns that can be anticipated and addressed. Examples are offered here that might provide helpful insights for demographers, statisticians, and disability advocates contemplating collection of data about disability in any community. However, a note of caution is also necessary: the study of disability cross-culturally is a recent endeavor and we have only begun to scratch the surface. There may be entirely new issues that arise as attempts are made to more accurately collect census data on disabled populations that have yet to be identified or even anticipated.

Finally, there are two main approaches to identifying individuals with a disability currently used in various regional and national censuses. The first is to use questions that simply identify the presence or absence of impairment in each individual. Such questions can be framed in a number of ways, but since at least the 18th century, in many countries, specific inquiries about whether any member of the household is blind or deaf, physically or intellectually impaired, or has mental health concerns, have been commonplace. A similar, but more general approach – asking if any respondent to a census or a member of their household has a disability, but not asking respondents to identify the exact nature of this disability – is less common, but also known. A second approach, based on the recent development of the International Classification of Impairment, Disability and Handicap (ICIDH), has eschewed the traditional classification by the type of impairment and instead concentrated on establishing measures of functional limitations. This new methodology allows census takers to collect more specific data on individuals with impairments within the population and is much less dependent on a medical model for defining disability. Because other papers in this series will go into greater depth about classificatory schemes and the

ICIDH, it will not be discussed in depth here. However, the presence of the new classificatory scheme is noted because there are social and cultural issues that arise in this methodology as well, that may also have a significant impact on data collection, as will be discussed below.

CONCEPTUALIZING DISABILITY

Research over the past several decades has clearly shown that "disability" is defined and conceptualized differently from one society to the next. This has complex social, cultural, economic, and political implications that will affect how different cultures define and count their citizens with disability (Groce & Zola, 1993; Ingstad & White, 1995).

Indeed, some languages lack a single word for disability. There will be words for specific types of disability (i.e., "the blind," "the deaf," and so forth) but not a single word – and not necessarily a single conceptual category – for a group that would include individuals with all types of impairments. There may be words grouping all who live with a disability into a larger category such as "the unfortunates" but these types of generic labels often include a wide range of individuals, many of whom would not in other situations, be considered disabled.

In such cases, even the words chosen for censuses must be carefully thought through. Asking about "the disabled" or inventing a new politically correct term to refer to those with a specific type of impairment, may result in vague or inaccurate answers from members of the community (UNICEF, 1999). In the United States, for example, while educators and advocates have abandoned the pejorative term "mental retardation" for more acceptable terms such as "intellectually challenged," the older term is still routinely used by the general public. Census takers would not get the demographic information needed to make accurate policy decisions if the term "mentally retarded" was not used. This is not to endorse the use of insensitive or objectionable terms or words, only to recommend field testing terms and phrases before they are used on regional and national censuses to ensure that people are being asked to respond to terms they understand.

To complicate matters still further, different terms may be used for the same type of impairment among members of different regions or between members of different ethnic or minority communities within the same region. This is all the more significant if a country has more than one national language or if there are a number of local languages into which a census must be translated.

Likewise, in some countries, censuses have used questions on health status as a proxy for disability. However, asking a respondent "is anyone in your family in poor health?" can be misleading. While this type of question may help to identify individuals who have various chronic illnesses, in many societies, individuals with disability are not necessarily seen as unwell. Having a disability may be seen as a human "condition" not a medical issue. In such cases, an individual who has a chronic debilitating disease, may be seen as 'sick' while a neighbor down the street who is intellectually disabled or a child in the neighborhood who has a hearing loss, may be considered perfectly healthy and not listed when the census taker comes to the door. Indeed, the United Nations has made this distinction; clearly stating that one can be both disabled and healthy. Again, how the issue of disability is conceptualized and framed in a given society will influence both the questions asked and the responses collected (Groce, 1999; United Nations, 1993).

THE ICIDH

The ICIDH and in more recent years the International Classification of Functioning, Disability and Health have been developed to help redefine how disability is conceptualized, providing richer and more comprehensive sources of information for policy makers and advocates. The ICIDH overcomes the problem of using broad diagnostic categories by concentrating on describing an individual's ability to function within the surrounding social and physical environment. In many countries, there has been a move to have census questions use "functioning" as a frame of reference. In general, framing issues in terms of functioning (i.e. does anyone in your household need help dressing themselves, does anyone in your household need assistance in feeding themselves?) provides a way to reframe categories that theoretically should allow census takers to collect data with a new level of specificity (World Health Organization, 2001).

However, the ICIDH is not fool proof and presents census takers with a new set of problems that must be anticipated and addressed. Most notably – while the ICIDH allows better definition of impairments in the context of the surrounding environment, it does not allow for differences that occur because of income, class or caste, even within the same ethnic or minority community, and there are some interactions between functional ability and culture that needs to be further explored.

For example, within the same community, there may be significant differences in what individuals with identical types of impairments may be able to do. These differences will not reflect the individual's level of functioning nor even the cultural beliefs and practices of the surrounding community, but rather the differences between the rich and the poor. For example, the ability of an individual to use the toilet independently may depend upon whether the person and his family are wealthy and have a toilet in the home or whether they are poor and must use an outhouse many yards from the backdoor or a communal bathhouse at the end of the street. The ability to cook for oneself may depend on whether an individual with a disability can turn on an electric stove or whether he or she must bring in firewood and stand over an open hearth. Indeed, in many cities around the world, an impoverished individual with a disability may be able to look out his or her window and actually see the distant mansion or high-rise apartment house where someone with an identical disability lives a very different life. A young man with a spinal cord injury in the slum may be unable to work, be unable to afford a wheelchair to allow him to move freely even within his household and be unable to use the neighborhood bathhouse. He may be wholly dependent on his parents and siblings. A young man with a comparable injury in the high rise may have a wheelchair, work on his computer either at home or in an office and have an accessible kitchen, bathroom, and bedroom at his disposal. Indeed, as the son of a wealthy family, he may be able to hire several attendants for round the clock assistance – thus creating jobs for able-bodied individuals as a result of his disability.

Likewise, census questions that attempt to collect data on disability by asking about the use of rehabilitation devices and aids, may have unanticipated limitations based on poverty, or on whether the individual lives in a rural or urban location. A question such as "does the individual with a disability use a wheelchair," makes assumptions about availability of funds, and accessibility of services. The middle class and rich will be more likely to acquire rehabilitation aids such as wheelchairs or hearing aids, than the poor. Access to centers and services that distribute such assistive devices are often far more available to individuals living in urban areas as opposed to rural areas. In poor, rural communities with no sidewalks and roads, particularly in uneven or hilly terrain, use of a wheelchair within the community (even if it is affordable), may be much more restricted than in a city with paved roads and accessible public transportation. In many societies where males are given preference to household resources, a poor family may hesitate to pay for rehabilitative services or assistive devises for females, even if they would be willing to pay for comparable services for males. Even in countries such as Canada and Great Britain where there are strong national health care schemes in place, research indicates that for a variety of reasons, poorer individuals with disability and individuals with disability from ethnic and minority community are less likely to be able to access such services (Altman, 1997; Branigan, Steward, Tardif, & Veltman, 2001; Kaplan, 1999).

Differences in cultural attitudes also can provide variables that will be reflected in data collection through the ICIDH methodology. In countries where there are distinct differences in assumptions and attitudes toward disability among different ethnic and minority communities, these differences may be reflected in the types of information about disability census takers are able to collect. An interesting example of how socio-cultural values can affect function is reported by Gannotti in her study of disabled children in Puerto Rico and Puerto Rican immigrants to the United States mainland (Gannotti & Handwerker, 2002). Gannotti observed that young Puerto-Rican children with various types of physical impairments were feeding themselves at a significantly later age than were their disabled Anglo peers. These children were no less capable of feeding themselves than the children from non-Puerto Rican families, but they were perceived by their mothers and the surrounding family members to be frail and in need of more "mothering." Mothers who allowed their disabled children to try to feed themselves at an earlier age were criticized by other adults within the Puerto Rican community for being harsh and unsympathetic. The cultural beliefs impacted the physical functioning of the child – a loving mother was defined as one who continued to provide extra help for her disabled child in basic tasks such as feeding and dressing for an extended period of time.

WHO ASKS THE QUESTIONS: CONSTRAINTS FACED BY CENSUS TAKERS

An equally significant variable is the nature of the identity of the census takers and what type of discussion about disability is considered socially acceptable within the social matrix in which they and their respondents exist. In many countries or regions, distinct beliefs about disability will frame what questions census takers will ask and what data policy makers believe they need. Collecting data that provides comparability between disabled populations at national levels, can be complicated if those designing national censuses do not have recourse to established international standards. Equally of concern is that fact that within a country, beliefs and attitudes about disability may differ from one region to another or from one ethnic group to the next. A question designed to be straightforward and unobtrusive at the national level may be considered problematic and intrusive in light of local beliefs and practices.

Data regarding those who have a disability must be collected – as all census data – either by sending a census taker into a community to ask people about the composition of their household, or by sending a form to the households to be filled out and returned by someone from that household. In either case, at its heart, this is an exchange between individuals – and as such, there is always the possibility that social and cultural factors will influence the information collected. The fact that disability has a strong cultural component makes the manner in which disability information is collected, of particular relevance.

Around the world, individuals with disability and their families face may kinds of stigma. Those planning for and collecting population and household data must be aware of (and familiar with) the local beliefs and traditions if useable data are to be collected. For example, in many societies, there are beliefs that individuals are born with a disability as a result of incest, evidence of some sin that a parent or ancestor has committed or as a sign of divine displeasure (Ingstad & White, 1995; Nicholls, 1992). In countries where the belief in reincarnation is strong, it is often believed that a person born with a disability is being punished for sins in a previous life (Marfo, Walker, & Charles, 1994; Marshall & Largo, 1999). The belief that an individual may acquire a disability later in life as a punishment for a sin or misdeed is also widespread.

Individuals born with a disability in such communities are often kept isolated by parents and families, fearful that they will bring disgrace or discredit on the entire family unit. These individuals may rarely or never leave the family compound, they are unlikely to attend school, and may rarely or never take part in community or religious events. Where the option is available, parents may be strongly encouraged to have their children institutionalized at birth or in early childhood. Neighbors living immediately next door may be unaware of the existence of such a disabled child or adult. In such societies, it is unlikely that families who have hidden disabled members for years will readily offer information about them to census takers who appear at their doors.

Where there is a considerable amount of stigma against individuals with disability and a reluctance or refusal to admit that there is a disabled member of a household, census takers may be unable to ascertain accurate information even when census data are collected privately at each household. Census takers are even less likely to collect accurate information when census data are collected at public meetings or in public gathering places. The respondent for the household may simply not list the individual with a disability, may list the family member but fail to report that the individual has a disability, or may report the individual in his or her household as being disabled, but be vague about the exact nature or extent of the disability. In such communities, individuals with disability will be unlikely to answer for themselves – or even come to the door of the family home.

The family's concerns may extend far beyond being ashamed or worried what the neighbors will think. Their reticence to respond may reflect a very real and accurate assessment of the implications that public awareness of a family's disabled member may have for the entire family unit. For example, in places where marriages must be arranged for all the children in a household, the presence of a sibling with disability may substantially lower the chances of arranging a good marriage for other siblings. In such cases, parents responding to the census taker are balancing the welfare of the disabled child with the well being of all their other children (UNICEF, 1999).

Indeed, the local census taker himself or herself may not be anxious to collect this information. For example, there is a common folk belief reported in both developed and developing societies that when people talk about a person with disability (even utter their name or look at them), it is possible that their next child to be born with a similar type of disability (Newman, 1969). In such instances, not only might a parent or relative hesitate to give information about a disabled member of their household, but the census taker might also hesitate to ask about or record the name of such an individual, fearing that their own next child would be "at risk."

Social and cultural issues extend beyond beliefs about disability. Researchers studying responses to both surveys and census have long known that individual characteristics of those collecting information in the community, such as race and gender will in many cases, have an impact on the information collected. The US Census Bureau for example, goes to great length to recruit census takers from ethnic and minority communities to help ensure that returns from specific communities are adequately represented. In countries with several or many local languages, census takers are often recruited for their ethnic or tribal affiliations as well as for their linguistic skills.

In societies where there are very distinct differences in caste or class, deep divisions between ethnic or tribal groups, or in communities where educational, economic, or occupational groups are deeply divided, the specific affiliation of a census taker may affect respondents' willingness to reveal an impairment in a family member. On the other hand, a census taker with a background more similar to the respondents might make the individuals providing information feel more comfortable or "at home" in providing such information. However, while it is often assumed that respondents will be more likely to provide accurate information to census takers who share similar ethnic or linguistic backgrounds, in fact, in some cases, family members of individuals with disability may be even more reticent about providing information to census takers who are from the same community or ethnic group. The reason for this would be a fear that the census taker would share what they learn with other members of the community.

WHO ANSWERS THE QUESTIONS – CONSTRAINTS FACED BY HOUSEHOLD INFORMANTS

In the previous section, it was noted that the collection of census data involves a dialog between at least two individuals – the census taker and the respondent for the family or household being surveyed. The background of the census taker is an important variable in how much and what type of information is collected – especially when sensitive issues, such as disability, are raised. No less important however is what member of a household is chosen or allowed to provide the family information.

Where there is a heavy stigma against individuals with disability, parents might be more reluctant to admit to the presence of a disabled child than would grandparents, uncles, or aunts. In societies where it is believed that traits are inherited entirely through women, mothers may be more likely to underreport the presence of a disabled child than would men. In cultures where men are thought to have primary responsibility for causing a child's disability, men will be more likely to underreport. Should a census be designed to specifically collect information on "functional limitations" particularly in societies where women are the ones who are responsible for feeding, dressing, toileting, and so forth, men may be less able than women to accurately answer the questions about how much actual help a family member needs to function on a daily basis.

BELIEFS ABOUT HOW THE DATA WILL BE USED

A basic question that must be asked – and one that can only be answered by actual fieldwork within the communities from which data are being collected, is "where do people believe the census data goes?" Understanding disability in the context of society is complex and it would be entirely wrong to assume that only shame or fear guides disclosure (or lack of disclosure) about individuals who have a disability. Often lack of disclosure reflects efforts to protect beloved members of the family. Where census data *actually* goes is irrelevant – people will respond to questions based on where they *think* the information they provide goes and whom they believe has the ability to see it. This is particularly true with sensitive topics, and in many societies, having a disability, as noted above, is considered a very sensitive topic.

This concern may not involve traditional beliefs about disability, but rather reflects local or national history of administrative decision-making and the rights of the individual. How authorities have used census or demographic information in the past will play a major role in the willingness of people to offer information in future census efforts. For example, in the Soviet Union, parents who gave birth to significantly disabled child were strongly encouraged or legally required to institutionalize their child as soon as the disability was diagnosed. Many parents lived in fear that the authorities would identify their child as disabled and insist that they be institutionalized. For that reason, reports indicate that many parents tried to hide their child's disability from the officials for as long as possible. The tradition of hiding a disabled child from the authorities in this case, is not a reflection of the fear of stigma, noted earlier, but an attempt by desperate parents to keep a child at home with the family. Times may have changed and rules about institutionalization may have been relaxed, but families in these countries are also keenly aware that should political climates change again, their child, once reported to authorities, would now be on the official roles. Immigrants from such countries have taken this caution about reporting disability to the authorities as they have traveled to new lands. For example, failure of eastern European immigrants to seek help for a disabled child or to report that child to census collectors have been reported from the United States and Canada (Groce & Zola, 1993).

Additionally, in a number of countries, there is a concern (often a realistic concern) that identification of an individual as having an impairment, may make that individual ineligible for rights or services guaranteed to the rest of the community. Authorities determining who is eligible to attend school or to vote may take an individual with disability (no matter what the disability might be) off the registration rolls. Individuals with disability may be denied the right to participate in religious ceremonies or to obtain a marriage license.

CONCLUSIONS AND RECOMMENDATIONS

Increasingly, attempts to enumerate the number of individuals with disability are appearing on censuses around the world. As noted above, there are a number of cultural issues that will influence and in many cases, impede how information on disability is collected. Moreover, because attitudes toward disability may differ markedly between different regions within the same country or between members of different ethnic and minority populations living side-by-side in the same community, collection and analyses if such data must be approached with caution. Issues of socio-economic status, class and caste may further complicate how well individuals with disability will function within their households and their communities. These issues are raised not to discourage the collection of data on individual and populations with disability, but to caution experts collecting this data that disability is a complex issue and one which must be approached with knowledge of social, economic, political, and cultural norms and expectations.

A good way to begin is for those planning to collect census information on disability to call upon the expertise and insights of disability advocates living within the societies from which they hope to collect data. These individuals with disability may be uniquely knowledgeable of the social and cultural limitations placed upon open discussion of disability within their communities. Placing individuals with disability on advisory and oversight boards for population and household census collection would yield significant benefits in all societies. Having people with disability work as census collectors would also yield significant insights. Do individuals with disability who are working as census collectors, collect more data about disability? Are individuals with disabled family members more forthcoming to disabled census collectors? It is not currently known, but is an area for future research.

Additionally, the very people who are responsible for designing and implementing local population and household censuses are an important source of insight. How do they themselves understand and talk about disability? What do they know about how disability is currently discussed in public. Asking those designing censuses or responsible for training census takers a straightforward question, such as "how do you and your friends talk about disability outside of the office?" could lead to important insights.

Understanding social and cultural attitudes and practices should help determine whether issues such as ethnicity, gender, and class of both census taker and households may influence the types of data gathered. Openness about disability or reticence to discuss the matter will also help determine whether information should be collected in a public forum, by household or in individual interviews – and with what member of the family. If census information is taken in an individual interview with a head of a household, or if a representative of the household is asked to fill out a form, then the amount of information gathered might be significantly more than if information is collected in a more public format. If a census is planned for a community or a specific ethnic or minority sub-population in which general discussion of disability is not the norm, then specific measures must be taken to determine what is the most culturally appropriate way to ask about this subject in the field.

Even here, it is important to anticipate the complexity of the social dynamics. Where there is significant cultural diversity within a country, having representatives with disability from one or more of the minority or ethnic communities in that society participate in planning for or collection of data, in addition to having a disabled representative from the main cultural group, could be very productive. Too often, representatives with disability are drawn only from the dominant ethnic or minority group and these representatives will be more likely to be male than female. Yet the amount of diversity within disabled populations argues strongly for using representatives from ethnic and minority groups, as well as women with disability, to round out the understanding that census takers will need to obtain truly accurate and representative information.

Again, it must be stressed that in order to collect meaningful data on disability within a population it is important to understand (and if it is unknown, to begin research) what the traditional local beliefs and attitudes are concerning disability. We do know that these beliefs are often very localized and may differ from one ethnic group to another – thus complicating census efforts that are designed to cover an entire region or provide national census data. For example, one tribal group or ethnic sub-population may forbid the open discussion or even "naming" of a person in the household with a disability; while members of a tribal group who live nearby may openly and freely discuss issues of disability in their families. (Indeed, in many parts of the world, drift into urban areas by families from many different ethnic and clan groups may mean that significantly different attitudes toward disability will be found in households in the same apartment building.) Finally, identification and discussion of disability in countries will depend on where people think the information will go and what it will be used for.

Insuring that all these issues are addressed will be difficult and time consuming. However, there are ways to anticipate many of these issues. Better research will help us understand more. However, even at this point, it is important to start with the understanding that we must be very careful about what we assume we know about disability in a cultural context. This is nowhere more important than when we attempt to develop and collect population and household census data.

Many of the issues raised are probably already familiar to census experts who have had to anticipate similar issues in other complex and diverse populations. The ultimate goal is to ensure that the information collected on individuals with disability reflect the actual numbers, status, and issues confronted by this large and largely overlooked population. Only then can policy makers appreciate the strength and anticipate the needs of those with disability in their communities.

REFERENCES

Altman, B. (1997). Does access to acute medical care imply access to preventive care: A comparison of women with and without disabilities. *Journal of Disability Policy Studies*, *8*(1–2), 99–128.

Branigan, M., Steward, D., Tardif, G., & Veltman, A. (2001). Perceptions of primary healthcare services among persons with physical disabilities, Part 2: Quality issues. *Medscape General Medicine*, *3*(2). http://www.medscape.com/viewarticle/408123.print

Gannotti, M., & Handwerker, W. P. (2002). Puerto Rican understandings of child disability: Methods for the cultural validation of standardized measures of child health. *Social Science & Medicine*, *55*(12), 11–23.

Groce, N., & Zola, I. K. (1993). Multiculturalism, chronic illness and disability. *Pediatrics*, *91*(5), 1048–1055.

Groce, N. (1999). Disability in a cross-cultural perspective: Rethinking disability. *The Lancet*, *354*, 756–757.

Ingstad, B., & White, S. (1995). *Disability and culture*. Berkeley: University of California Press.

Kaplan, L. (1999). Community-based services in the United States: A pediatric perspective. *The Lancet*, *354*, 761–762.

Marfo, K., Walker, S., & Charles, P. (Eds) (1994). *Childhood disability in developing countries*. New York: Praeger.

Marshall, C., & Largo, H. (1999). Disability and rehabilitation: A context for understanding the American Indian experiences. *The Lancet*, *354*, 750–760.

Newman, L. (1969). Folklore of pregnancy: Wives' tales in contra costa county, California. *Western Folklore*, *28*(2), 112–135.

Nicholls, R. (1992). An examination of some traditional African attitudes towards disability. *Traditional and changing views of disability in developing societies*. Monograph #53. Durham, NH: National Institute of Disability and Rehabilitation Research.

UNICEF. (1999). *An overview of young people living with disabilities: Their needs and their rights*. New York: UNICEF Inter-Divisional Working Group on Young People, Programme Division.

United Nations. (1993). *Standard rules on the equalization of opportunities for persons with disabilities. General Assembly Resolution 48/96. December 1993*. New York: United Nations.

World Health Organization. (2001). *International classification of functioning, disability and health*. Geneva: WHO.

REFLECTIONS ON DISABILITY LANGUAGE AND THE ICIDH/ICF

Yerker Andersson

ABSTRACT

The following is a reaction to the new developments in measurement language and the approaches to definitions of disability developed through the revisions of the ICIDH and the resulting ICF. It provides the view of an individual who has lived with limitations as well as an individual who has served as the president of an international disability organization.

I have been thinking about the effect the ICIDH[1] and its later version the ICF[2] have had on language usage relating to disability. The ICIDH made several significant changes in the vocabularies about disability used by different languages. The ICIDH conceptualized three categories or aspects: impairment, disability and handicap. "Impairment" and "disability" were used as substitutes for references to the individual in place of the old and now disliked term "handicapped" or its equivalent in many countries (even though "handicapped" still is tolerable in a few countries (including my native country, Sweden)). Handicap as conceptualized by the ICIDH was now a reference to the environment rather than the individual. Some national and international disability organizations adopted either "disability" or "disabled" as terminology instead of "handicap" or "handicapped,"

International Views on Disability Measures: Moving Toward Comparative Measurement
Research in Social Science and Disability, Volume 4, 55–60

ISSN: 1479-3547/doi:10.1016/S1479-3547(05)04005-4

respectively. For example, in 1992 the World Federation of the Deaf and the International Federation of Hard of Hearing rejected the general term "hearing impaired" in favor of the older terms "deaf" and "hard of hearing." However, the term "impairment" was retained by other disability groups. For example, "mobility impairment" is preferred by wheelchair users. Additionally, the World Blind Union uses "visually impaired" and "blind," and Inclusion International still uses the term "mental impairment." According to laws in several countries, "blind" has usually been applied to all those whose vision could vary from totally lost to severely limited. But those whose vision is not totally lost prefer to be called visually impaired, not blind. While most of those wearing hearing aids usually are classified as "hearing impaired," most of those wearing eyeglasses were not necessarily regarded as visually impaired. It must be noted, however, that this terminology remains ambiguous. For example, persons with tunnel vision who have been permitted to drive a car, are able to read but with some difficulty.

The term "people with disabilities" has consistently been employed in US government policies and other documents. "Disabled people" – as a term – has been avoided in US government policies and several disability organizations. However, "disabled people" was acceptable in Great Britain in both legislative policies and publications. "Survivor" now is used by landmine victims and individuals with mental illness. These different uses of disability vocabulary suggest a degree of disagreement about the appropriate use of the ICIDH terms "disability," "impairment" and "handicap" in the disability community.

It might be worth noting that questions about vocabulary have also been raised when referring to those who would not be identified as having a disability. The phrases "people without disabilities" or "with no disabilities" or "non-disabled individuals" are no longer acceptable as a terminology. The chair of DISTAB (Disability Tabulations) proposed using the phrase "with no reportable disabilities." This is an approach I was willing to accept. The National Council on Disability dropped these terms when I argued that virtually all human beings would have more or fewer physical, sensory or mental limitations or shortcomings which some might label as disabilities depending on societal demands. For example, hand cramps as a result of computer use now has been regarded as a disability by US courts evaluating the eligibility for disability benefits, but not so in countries where computers are not easily available. Disagreements of this nature have appeared in recent debates on the internet (the website http://disability-awareness@yahoogroups.com) during 2002.

However, the disability community is in full agreement that disability should not be viewed as an exclusively medical phenomenon. Several disability organizations have repeatedly asserted that individuals with disabilities can be as healthy as – or even healthier than – people with no reportable disabilities.

T. Bedirhan Üstün et al. have acknowledged in their reply to David Pfeiffer's article "The ICIDH and the Need for its Revision" (1998, p. 520)[3], that it is a mistake to treat "all aspects of disablement phenomena" as a purely medical problem (1998, p. 829)[4]. Many countries around the world have for a long time, use normalcy as a criterion for measuring the permanent or unusual limitations, shortcomings or incapacities of individuals as parts of human life or health, instead of accepting diversity. On the other hand, as Üstün et al. state, "the vast proportion of persons with a disability around the world have chronic disease conditions that require and often do not receive adequate medical [and rehabilitative] treatments" (1998, p. 829). This is a fact that the disability community cannot deny. However, medical or rehabilitative treatments are not the only paths to recovery. The importance of support groups and environmental factors facilitating health recovery and maintenance – a view shared by not only the disability community but also health professionals, especially those favoring the holistic approach – has not been acknowledged as equal in importance to, or in addition to, health treatments in many countries yet.

In his article "The ICIDH and the Need for its Revision," David Pfeiffer, expresses his belief that the ICIDH and ICIDH-2 (now ICF) "are dangerous and must be dealt with by the community of people with disabilities." (1998, p. 520). In reply to this warning, Üstün et al. assert that "persons with disabilities and their international and local organisations have been active[ly] in" (1998, p. 829) the preparation of ICF. An examination of Pfeiffer's bibliography and citations suggests that he has relied mostly on the views of scholars who have disabilities. The views of those organizations of people with disabilities and individuals with disabilities consulted by WHO might have been different from those of scholars or researchers with disabilities. But the assumption that scholars who have disabilities can be the only spokespersons for the disability world suggests some degree of elitism or paternalism. Instead, those scholars should perhaps share their criticisms with appropriate organizations of people with disabilities; those organizations could then update and publicize their views or could issue new policies in the same way other scholars and researchers share their views with lawmakers, government officials and policy makers.

Obviously, the involvement of disability scholars in the development and management of research projects should still be encouraged, because such a diversity is needed for their analytical and interpretation skills. Fortunately, this involvement, best known as Participatory Action in Research or PAR, has recently been adopted in health research. Following this trend, the first ICIDH revision meeting endorsed the principle that persons with disabilities should be involved in the revision process as early as 1993. (Dr. Paul Placek – personal communication). Without the involvement of both organizations of people with disabilities and disability scholars, the WHO team would probably have been less willing to adopt both the social and medical models of disability than prior to the publication of ICIDH.

The Americans with Disabilities Act and similar laws or policies in Europe (see Mužoz & de Lorenzo, 1997)[5] and other countries interpret disability as a limitation or interference with daily activities such as walking, seeing, hearing, etc. At the same time these laws propose modifications in environmental factors such as the societal understanding of sensory, physical and mental capabilities; architectural and transportation designs; the accessibility of mass media and others. As history suggests, interaction among organizations of people with disabilities and human rights advocates, including lawyers, and scholars have exerted much influence on this legal evolution (National Council on Disability, 1997)[6].

As the emergence of ICF is a relatively new international event, it may be too early to find out what views the community of people with disabilities have toward it. Based on discussions with both international disability leaders and individuals with disabilities at international meetings, and based upon articles from different perspectives on disabilities in periodicals, and research findings, let me describe a few possible implications of the new conceptualization of disability.

Having participated in several meetings of DISTAB, an international workgroup which seeks to backcode survey questions to ICF codes, I have the impression that the measurement of disability, as implemented by DISTAB, is promising because it may yield much more internationally comparable data than in the past. Previously the numbers of persons with sensory, physical and mental limitations have been reported, with emphasis on medical categories. The new approach with a focus on daily activities – such as hearing, seeing, walking, as well as the inclusion of the use of hearing aids, sign language interpreting services, braille services, wheelchairs, etc. will, for the first time, provide information about the degree of participation in society. For example, understanding the use of hearing aids and interpreting or captioning services in a given country would begin to improve the involvement of deaf and hard of hearing individuals in social life. Knowledge of the number of wheelchair users could be used as an indicator of the level of freedom to move around in meeting rooms or on transportation. The effects of participation and isolation have repeatedly been discussed as health improvement factors in sociology and psychology. This new approach will certainly require a high level of teamwork among not only health professionals but also the governments, parliaments, architects, designers and disability advocates. It is consistent with the Draft of ICIDH-2's shift from "a 'consequence of disease' classification to a 'components of health' classification."

However, this new word "activities" might be untranslatable in some countries and hence might cause some difficulties in the ability to measure disability in those countries. Fortunately, the members of DISTAB and other research teams have been developing and comparing the new measures of disability in different languages, which should certainly lead to a clearer concept of "activities." As far as I know, the concept of "activities" has not appeared yet in laws granting equality or banning discrimination in many countries (Mužoz & de Lorenzo, 1997).

As recently as 1999, in a meeting organized by the Organization of American States, a group of government delegates spent about 3/4th of their entire meeting time on the attempt to find a better definition of "disability" for their review of a proposed policy forbidding discrimination on the ground of disability. For this reason, they were unable to reach a consensus at the end of their two-day meeting. No doubt, the definition of disability only in terms of body functions and structure will never be satisfactory in the future. All human beings have at least one limitation on their mental, sensory or physical capabilities, which may be more or less tolerable depending on societal or cultural demands. These limitations can either emerge or disappear as disabilities whenever societal or technological changes occur. For example, a former teacher of mine would have been considered as an individual with disability in our computer age as he had some difficulties in dialing phone calls and, therefore, would not be able to acquire typing or computer skills, now a common requirement in several professional occupations. Obesity is another good example as it is appreciated in some countries and not tolerable in others.

In conclusion, ICF in general is a great improvement of ICIDH but cannot be expected to be a perfect classification of health or disability. Revisions will certainly appear in later editions. For example, the English-speaking deaf community will likely react to the inappropriate use of "formal sign language" in the English version of ICF because it presumes that only formal signs should be expected to be used for everyday conversation. Such an expectation, of course, is absurd. Oddly enough, the Spanish version uses "lengue de signos conventional" and the French version the plain but most appropriate term "langue des signes." Any attempt by health professionals, government officials and lawmakers to develop a better understanding of health, or disability without a consideration of the current views of different groups and new modifications in social, attitudinal and physical factors will likely reduce the usefulness of ICF and its future successors. Individuals with a cochlear implant may still consider themselves as deaf persons, rather than hearing, not only because the quality of their hearing cannot be comparable to that of unassisted hearing but also because sign language has for a long time existed as a part of their daily life. Organizations of the deaf in several countries have already announced that individuals with a cochlear implant would still be eligible for full membership. On the other hand, those having received a laser treatment for their eyes apparently believe that they no longer are visually impaired. Such new differences exist not only between people with disabilities but also within each disability.

In its measure of disability, ICF now includes activities, environmental factors and participation, in addition to body functioning and structural and personal factors, so it now requires a multi-disciplinary approach to disability studies. This expansion will certainly make information about people with disabilities and no reportable disabilities more reliable and more useful for government officials, health professionals, lawmakers and industrialists. In the long run, the measurements of body functions, activities, participation and environmental factors must, however, be designed so that its findings can satisfy the needs of different human groups, not only the disability community.

NOTES

1. ICIDH. (1980). *International classification of impairments. Disabilities, and handicaps*. Geneva: World Health Organization.
2. ICF. (2001). *International classification of functioning, disability and health*. Geneva: World Health Organization.
3. Pfeiffer, D. (1998). The ICIDH and the need for its revision. *Disability & Society*, *13*(4), 503–523.
4. Üstün, T. B., Bickenbach, J., Badley, E., & Chatterji, S. (1998). A reply to David Pfeiffer "The ICIDH and the need for its revision." *Disability & Society*, *13*(5), 829–831.
5. Mužoz, S. M., & de Lorenzo, R. (Eds). (1997). *European disability law*. Madrid: Escuela Libre Editorial.
6. National Council on Disability. (1997). *Equality of opportunity: The making of the Americans with disabilities act*. Washington, DC, July 26.

SECTION II:
COUNTRY SPECIFIC EXPERIENCES

REVIEW OF PRACTICES IN LESS DEVELOPED COUNTRIES ON THE COLLECTION OF DISABILITY DATA☆

Angela Me and Margaret Mbogoni

ABSTRACT

The aim of the paper is to review the experiences of developing countries in collecting disability data with regard to the methods and definitions used. The review is based on data in the United Nations Disability Statistics Database, version 2 (DISTAT-2). We analyze the prevalence rates of disability in relation to the characteristics of questions used to identify persons with disabilities and the relationship between disability prevalence and other social and economic indicators. The wide difference in approaches used by countries to identify persons with disabilities result in very different rates of disability prevalence, thus making the comparison

☆The analysis is limited to the experience of the countries classified as "developing countries" in the UN classification of macro geographical (continental) regions, geographical sub-regions, and selected economic and other groupings (http://unstats.un.org/unsd/methods/m49/m49regin.htm). The views presented in this paper are those of the authors and not necessarily those of the United Nations.

International Views on Disability Measures: Moving Toward Comparative Measurement
Research in Social Science and Disability, Volume 4, 63–87

ISSN: 1479-3547/doi:10.1016/S1479-3547(05)04006-6

of these rates very problematic. The paper gives suggestions on how to improve methods to collect data on disability.

CONCEPTUALIZATION OF DISABILITY

The way disability is conceptualized and viewed has radically changed in the last 30 years. In the past the "Old Paradigm" was based on a medical model that looked at disability as an "unwanted" condition where people with disabilities were not expected to play a social role (Pfeiffer, 2001). Disability was seen exclusively as an individual characteristic and was described in terms of pathologies such as blindness, deafness, paralysis, and mental retardation, conditions that are located within the individual. Several social movements changed these views and developed new interpretations (Pfeiffer, 2001) where the experience of persons with disabilities is defined in all its complexity with a shift from the focus on the individual to the predominant role of the society and the environment. Different conceptual models have been developed to elaborate the relationship. The Nagi model (1965) developed first and more recently the International Classification of Functioning, Disability and Health (ICF) (WHO, 2001)[1] set a milestone in the description of the disablement process. Both models consider disability as a group of related concepts describing the consequences of a health condition in an interaction with a person's environment, on the individual body, individual activities and overall participation of the individual in the society (Jette & Badley, 2000; IOM, 2002).

The ICF has modeled a new paradigm by conceptualizing disability as a multidimensional construct. Rather than restricting disability within narrow biomedical or social models the ICF has identified all major dimensions in an integrated bio-psycho-social model. Such a model strongly advocates the integration of the environment that the disability experience takes place in. Unlike most disability models, the ICF does not restrict disability to a minority status that belongs to a small sub-set of the society with certain bodily impairments. The ICF, like the IOM, takes a "universal model" that expands the examination of functioning onto the total human experience and tries to capture the full spectrum of life.

The recognition of the role of the environment brings new challenges to the measurement of disability. The description of the medical model was, from a measurement point of view, an easier task. It involved the static dichotomy of having or not having a certain condition. In the new frameworks such as the ICF model, disability is seen more as a continuum where different domains and degrees of experiences are to be considered. The measurement of different points in this continuum requires the development of new instruments carefully designed to identify the range of persons with disabilities from those who have very severe types of disability to those who have more mild disabilities.

DEFINITIONS OF DISABILITY USED IN DEVELOPING COUNTRIES

Annex 1 gives examples of definitions of disability used in national population censuses. As can be seen from these examples, disability is diversely defined in different countries, thereby making generalizations among them difficult. Different conceptual models are implied by these definitions. While some countries define disability exclusively in terms of medical conditions, – "physical or mental disorder" or a "deformity or deficient functioning of any limb" (Aruba, Pakistan, Sri Lanka, and Morocco), others define it in terms of the ability to perform ("do") activities (Zambia, Philippines, Nigeria, West Bank, and Gaza). Few countries defined disability in a social context making reference to participation in domains such as education, work, and household activities (Bahamas, Cyprus, Poland, and Uganda). In some cases, definitions make reference to a "norm" and persons with disability are defined as limited in performing what is considered "normal" (Bahamas, Uganda, Philippines, and Nigeria).

DIFFICULTIES WITH TRANSLATING DEFINITIONS INTO QUESTIONS

In general, the definition used sets the scope of who is targeted and determines the type of data that are collected. However, one of the biggest challenges countries face in the collection of disability data is the translation of definitions into questions (Altman, 2001). As some of the examples of definitions show, some countries have made great progress in the conceptualization of disability by adopting definitions that are close to the ICF or its predecessor, the International Classification of Impairments, Disabilities and Handicaps (ICIDH). However, looking at the measures used to identify persons with disabilities, difficulties have been experienced in including the concepts in the definitions into questions. Often the importance of designing questions to identify persons with disabilities according to these concepts has been underestimated. As an example, definitions using a social approach to disability have not always been converted to questions that reflect this perspective. In many developing countries, particularly in Africa and in Latin America, the questions used to identify persons with disabilities are of the type: "Is there anybody in the household who is disabled?" This question has a different meaning depending on the cultural interpretation of what is considered as a disability that conceivably varies from country to country (Groce, 1999).

Table 1 compares the definitions with the related questions used in the censuses of three of the countries presented in Annex 1. As it can be noted, the questions used do not necessarily encompass the definition used. For example, in Nigeria, disability is defined in terms of ability to carry out everyday life activities by the person and yet the question used targets only severe impairments, including being blind, deaf, crippled, and mentally retarded.

Socio-Cultural Determinants

There are also several cultural aspects that affect the measurement of disability. In many countries disability is stigmatized and this makes the identification of persons with disabilities more challenging. One of the greatest problems reported globally by experts and persons with disabilities is prejudice (UNICEF, 1999). This causes people to be reluctant to admit the presence of a person with disability in the household and interviewers tend to not ask about disability unless a person with a very severe kind of disability is seen during the interview. Unfortunately, the wording of disability questions has not always encouraged a positive or even a neutral reaction of respondents and interviewers.

Disability is also often perceived only as a medical and "visible" concern. Sometimes, enumerators fill in answers to disability questions on the basis of observation. An example is the following instruction included in a census questionnaire: "Ask this question only if there is in the household a disabled person".

THE EFFECT OF QUESTION FORM AND CONTENT ON THE PREVALENCE RATE OF DISABILITY: EVIDENCE FROM NATIONAL EXPERIENCES

The wide range of disability rates reported by less developed countries is due to several factors that include:

- Differences in experiences of disability including, the prevalence of chronic diseases and availability of medical interventions, as well as societal perceptions and attitudes.
- Differences in definitions of disability.

Table 1. Comparison of Definitions and Questions used to Identify Persons with Disabilities in Selected Countries.

Country	Definition	Question
Nigeria, census 1991	Disability has been defined as a restriction or lack (resulting from an impairment) of ability to perform an activity in the manner or within the range considered normal for a human being. Disability is characterized by excesses or deficiencies of customarily expected activity performance and behavior, and these may be temporary or permanent, reversible or irreversible, and progressive or regressive. Disabilities may arise as a direct consequence of impairment or as a response by the individual, particularly psychologically, to a physical, sensory, or other impairment. Disability represents objectification of an impairment, and as such if reflects disturbances at the level of the person. Therefore, disability is concerned with abilities, in the form of composite activities and behaviors, that are generally accepted as essential components of everyday life	*Nature of disability*: 1. Not disabled 2. Deaf 3. Dumb 4. Deaf and dumb 5. Blind 6. Crippled 7. Mentally retarded/ lunatic 8. Others, specify
Philippines, census 1990	Disability refers to any restriction or lack (resulting from an impairment) of ability to perform an activity in the manner or within the range considered normal for a human being	Does…have any total and permanent physical or mental disability?
Uganda, census 1991	A disability is defined as any condition that prevents a person from living normal social and working life	Is anyone who was in the household on census night disabled? Yes/No Nature of disability: blind, mentally ill, deaf and dumb, polio, amputee, leprosy, cripple, lame, epilepsy, mentally retarded, other

- Different methodologies used in the measurement of disability, including the type of question(s) asked, the choice of respondent (self vs proxy reporting), method of data collection (survey or census), and the mode of data collection (face-to-face interview, mail-back questionnaire, telephone interview, etc.).
- The range and types of impairments or disabilities included in the question.

For purposes of this paper, we have limited ourselves to the effect of question content and wording on the prevalence rates. To accomplish this, we reviewed some studies carried out in developing countries to understand what the types of questions used to identify persons with disabilities are, what the impact of different questions on the prevalence of disability is, and to highlight some of the problems related to the comparison of disability data among developing countries. This review is based on information available in the United Nations Disability Statistics Database, version 2 (DISTAT-2) published in 2001.[2]

Information in the database shows that the data collected by developing countries on persons with disabilities has increased significantly in the past few decades. Data on prevalence rates by age, sex, study, and type of data collection and questions used in national studies to measure disability, from DISTAT-2, is available on the Internet at: http://unstats.un.org/unsd/demographic/sconcerns/disability/disab2.asp.

DISTAT-2 was published in 2001 and covers 111 national studies on disability carried out in 78 countries across all regions of the world. The data included in the database are those reported by countries. Of the 111 studies in DISTAT-2, 65 represent population censuses, 44 are sample surveys, and the rest are based on administrative sources. The breakdown of the 93 studies carried out in developing countries by type and region is presented in Table 2. In many developing countries, particularly in Africa, Asia, and to some extent South America, the population census is the only source of data on disability.

There are substantial differences among developing countries in the rates of disability prevalence, and if compared with developed countries, these rates seem to be lower on average. Disability rates[3] in less developed

Table 2. Disability Data Collection in Developing Countries by Source of Data.

Source of Data	Africa	Asia	Caribbean	Latin America	Europe	Total
Total	38	33	7	12	3	93
Censuses	29	22	7	8	3	69
Surveys	9	11	0	4	0	24

countries vary from 0.17% to 9.86% with 59 countries that have rates below 2%, 18 countries from 2% to 4% and 11 countries that have prevalence rates greater than 4%. Other countries such as Australia, Canada, The Netherlands, United States, and New Zealand have rates that range from 11.6% to 20%. We would argue that the main factors that influence the high degree of variation among developing countries and between developing and developed countries is due to differences in how disability is defined and measured.

The high degree of variation in definitions of disability and of screening strategies used is also cited as a major cause of the observed differences in the crude disability rates for 55 countries in the first version of DISTAT which was published in 1988 (United Nations, 1990; Chamie, 1989).

Using data from countries where information on methods was available in the database, we analyzed the relationships between different question designs used and prevalence rates obtained with the idea of measuring performance of different typologies of questions to identify persons with disabilities.

Looking at the measures used to identify the persons with disabilities, we considered the following factors:

- To whom is the question addressed? Is it household-based or person-based?[4]
- Is the question based on a list of impairments?
- Does the measure include a single question or multiple questions?
- Is mental disability specifically mentioned in the wording of the question?
- Is the measure cognitively simple or complex?
- Are the words "disability" or "handicap" mentioned in the wording of the question?
- Is the measure based on activity limitations?

All the measures used to identify persons with disabilities were classified on the basis of these characteristics converted into dichotomous variables. Differences in prevalence of disability were then analyzed in relation to the use of characteristics in terms of comparison of prevalence rates and analysis of variance (ANOVA).

After having carryed out one-way ANOVA (Type III) studies to analyze the effect of the above-mentioned question characteristics into the disability prevalence rates, only two of the seven question characteristics showed a statistically significant impact on the reporting of disability:

- To whom the question is addressed, i.e., person level or household level question. The analysis shows that a person-based question identifies on average 2.3% of population as having disabilities while a household-based question identifies only 1.6%.

- Question based/not based on a list of impairments. Questions not based on a specific list of impairments seem to have higher reported levels of disability than questions based on a generic question. Measures based on a limited set of impairments identify on average 1.4% of persons with disabilities while measures not based on a limited set identify 2.6%.

The significant impact of these two characteristics was confirmed also when we performed different hierarchical ANOVA to look at the net effect of all the question characteristics on the prevalence rate. The hierarchical analysis confirmed that significant effect of the person/household question and of the questions based on a list of impairments. In addition, another characteristic, *the use of single/multiple questions*, showed a significant effect. Tables 3 and 4 show the effect of the three significant factors[5] into two different hierarchical decompositions of the total disability rate.

Looking at extremely low (<1%) compared to higher (>3%)[6] prevalence rates, the same two characteristics have a significant impact.[7] A person-based question is for example 5 times more likely to have a prevalence rate >3 than a household-based question while a question not based on a set of impairments is 9.7 times as likely to produce a prevalence rate >3 as a question based on a set of impairments.

Studying the impact of different types of measures used to identify elderly persons with disabilities, features that seem to have a significant impact on generating high prevalence rates (>10%) are: *person-based questions, the word disability is not mentioned, questions based on activity limitations*, and question is *not based on a limited list of impairments*. We found no significant effects of any of the characteristics considered on the prevalence rates of children.

Table 3. Analysis of Variance of Total Prevalence Rate, Hierarchical Decomposition.

	Sum of Squares	Mean Square	*F*	Sig.	Observed Power
Intercept	270.11	270.11	5.79	0.12	0.32
Household/person-based	11.02	11.02	5.15	0.03	0.61
Single/multiple questions	13.23	13.23	5.16	0.03	0.58
List of impairments	21.58	21.58	3.10	0.23	0.18

Note: The table is based on an ANOVA Type I. The purpose is to study the effect of the listed question characteristics on the prevalence rate in a hierarchical way. The effect of the first characteristic (household/person-based) is first analyzed adjusting for the effect of the other, below listed characteristics. Taking as threshold a significance level of 0.05, the effect of household/person-based questions and single/multiple questions show a significant effect on the prevalence rate.

Table 4. Analysis of Variance of Total Prevalence Rate, Hierarchical Decomposition.

	Sum of Squares	Mean Square	*F*	Sig.	Observed Power
Intercept	270.11	270.11	6.55	0.21	0.18
List of impairments	39.50	39.50	18.46	0.00	0.99
Household/person-based	5.87	5.87	1.98	0.19	0.25
Single/multiple questions	0.46	0.46	0.03	0.89	0.05

Note: The table is based on an ANOVA Type I. The purpose is to study the effect of the listed question characteristics on the prevalence rate in a hierarchical way. The effect of the first characteristic (question based on a list of impairments) is first analyzed adjusting for the effect of the other, below listed characteristics. Taking as threshold a significance level of 0.05, the effect of questions based on a list of impairments show a significant effect on the prevalence rate.

While performing the ANOVA to study the effect of question characteristics the different methods of data collection (census, survey) and regions were always taken in consideration. Performing the ANOVA to study the effect of method of data collection and region, no significant results were found.

The Different Case of the Caribbean

Some Caribbean countries that are included in DISTAT-2 show a common pattern of disability rates that is different if compared with other regions. Aruba, Belize, Bermuda, and Saint Vincent and the Grenadines used very different types of questions[8] but they all obtained high prevalence rates (from 5.5% to 7.6%) in comparison to other countries that used similar types of questions. The commonality they have is that they all used person-based questions. It would be interesting to look into the cultural dimensions of disability in the Caribbean to see if the high reporting is due to a common understanding of disability that is different from other developing countries.

TO WHAT EXTENT ARE COUNTRIES USING THE ICF IN THEIR DATA COLLECTION ON DISABILITY?

Current national practices in disability measurement sometimes make it difficult to classify disability studies according to the three major ICF classification domains (Body Functions and Structures, Activities and Participation, Environmental Factors) (Mbogoni, 2003). Although definitions could give an indication of the way disability measurement is approached – sometimes there are inconsistencies between definitions and the approaches used in the screening questions and between questions and types of disability considered. Table 1 included examples of different approaches used in definitions and questions; Table 5 shows examples of different approaches used between questions and the description of types of disabilities. As it is showed in the two examples in Table 5, sometimes the types of disability describe more than one domain of disability and in some cases diseases are included on the same list as types of disabilities. This leads not only to difficulties in the classification of the studies according to a single disability domain, but may also mislead the interpretation of the results. The impairments for example that are described in the types of disabilities of the 2002 census of Uganda refer only to the people who reported activity limitations.

For most of the developing countries included in DISTAT-2, the questions are impairment based but not strictly related to either the ICIDH or its revised version, the ICF. Information in DISTAT version 1 presented in the Disability Statistics Compendium (United Nations, 1990) and analyzed by Chamie (1989) also shows that in most studies, persons with disabilities were identified through the use of an impairment screen (United Nations, 1990).

The types of disabilities collected in censuses and surveys vary greatly from country to country. Of the 64 studies for which a question is available in DISTAT-2, half (31 studies), mainly in Africa, investigated disability through a checklist of impairments. This approach was used mainly in population censuses. The following is an example of a checklist of severe impairments used in a 1991 census of Nigeria – Nature of disability: (a) not disabled; (b) deaf; (c) dumb; (d) deaf and dumb; (e) blind; (f) crippled; (g) mentally retarded/lunatic; and (h) others.

Some developing countries are moving toward activity limitations to describe the types of disabilities. In the 2000 round of censuses for example countries such as Bahamas, Belize, Jamaica, Mauritius, West Bank and Gaza, and Trinidad and Tobago considered activities that included: seeing, hearing, speaking, moving/mobility, gripping, and learning.

Being a new classification, there is not much experience in the implementation of the ICF in data collection activities. However, there are some instances where it has been applied in developing countries. The World Health Organization, through its survey program, the *WHO Survey on Health and Health System Responsiveness*, has developed questions to assess functioning based on selected categories of the ICF.[9] These surveys have been carried out in 30 developing countries. The earlier questions on disability covered 19 categories[10] the current questionnaire 8 domains.

Table 5. Comparison of ICF Domains in Questions used to Identify Persons with Disabilities and in the Description of Types of Disabilities in Selected Countries.

Country	Question	Types of Disabilities
Uganda, census 2002	Does (name) have any difficulty moving, seeing, hearing, speech, or learning, which has lasted 6 months or more? *ICF domain: activity*	*Body functions*: 1. Limited use of legs 2. Limited use of arms 3. Hearing difficulty 4. Deafness 5. Poor vision 6. Blindness 7. Serious speech impediment 8. Dumb 9. Mental retardation *Disease*: 10. Mental illness 11. Epileptic 12. Rheumatism 13. Serious problem with back spine
South Africa, census 2001	Does (the person) have any serious disability that prevents his/her full participation in life activities (such as education, work, social life)? *ICF domain: participation*	*Body functions*: 1. Sight (blind/severe visual limitation) 2. Hearing (deaf, profound hard of hearing) 3. Communication (speech impairment) *Activity*: 1. Intellectual (serious difficulties in learning) 2. Emotional (behavioral, psychological) *Body structure/need assistive devices*: 4. Physical (e.g. needs wheelchair, crutches or prosthesis, limb, hand usage limitations)

Another application of the ICF is in the Level of Living Conditions Survey 2001 being conducted in Namibia and Zimbabwe by SINTEF Unimed – Health and Rehabilitation, a research group in Norway that is presented elsewhere in this volume.

ANALYSIS OF DISABILITY RATES IN DEVELOPING COUNTRIES IN RELATION TO OTHER SOCIAL AND ECONOMIC VARIABLES

Literature shows a relationship between disability and socio-economic development although this relationship is complex with no one clear direction of causality. It has been suggested, for instance, that the disability rate is a socio-economic indicator – a type of poverty index, or index of development (United Nations, 1990). Lower socio-economic status and higher poverty levels are associated with higher disability rates, e.g., higher illiteracy rates, poor nutritional status, lower immunization coverage of children, low birth weight of babies, higher unemployment rates, and lower occupational mobility.

Considering this linkage we analyzed the relationship between the disability prevalence rates included in DISTAT-2 and other social and economic variables such as nutrition, immunization, mortality, and economic wealth. The purpose of the analysis is to see if the data support these linkages. If the empirical data do not show a relationship between disability and social-economic development, we would argue that the problem lays with the different quality of disability data reflected in the different methodology used. The lack of uniform standards affects the quality of the data and hampers the comparison among countries.

From the UN system common database (http://unstats.un.org/unsd/default.htm), we selected the following four variables: life expectancy, GDP (measured as per capita GDP in international $PPP), percentage of children one year old immunized against measles, and percentage of children under five moderately or severely underweight. We analyzed the relationship between these social-economic variables and the prevalence of disability looking at correlation and regression models and factor analysis. The purpose of these analyses was to look for possible statistical relationships between disability prevalence and the other social-economic variables.

The results show the following:

- There are significant linear correlations between the social and economic indicators selected however, there are no significant correlations between prevalence of disability and all the other variables (see Table 6);

Table 6. Correlation Analysis between Social and Economic Variables and Disability Prevalence Rates.

	Life Expectancy	GDP Per Capita	Immunization	Malnutrition	Disability Prevalence
Life expectancy					
Pearson correlation	1	0.596*	0.515*	−0.535*	0.168
Sig. (2-tailed)	—	0.000	0.000	0.000	0.124
GDP per capita					
Pearson correlation	0.596*	1	0.341*	−0.402*	0.176
Sig. (2-tailed)	0.000	—	0.003	0.000	0.125
Immunization					
Pearson correlation	0.515*	0.341*	1	−0.517*	0.153
Sig. (2-tailed)	0.000	0.003	—	0.000	0.175
Malnutrition					
Pearson correlation	−0.535*	−0.402	−0.517*	1	−0.090
Sig. (2-tailed)	0.000	0.000	0.000	—	0.426
Disability prevalence					
Pearson correlation	0.168	0.176	0.153	−0.90	1
Sig. (2-tailed)	0.124	0.125	0.175	0.426	—

*Significant at the 0.01 level (2-tailed).

- Looking at linear regression models, none of the social-economic variables significantly predicts the trend of disability prevalence (when considering prevalence rate as the dependent variable) and vice versa, disability rates do not give any significant contribution to the prediction trend of all the other variables (nutrition, GDP, mortality, and immunization), when considering prevalence rate as one of the independent variables;
- Looking at factor analysis it appears that social and economic variables are all related to a single factor that we could interpret as related to a social-economic component while disability prevalence is associated with a different dimension that cannot be associated with the social and economic environment of a country (and therefore cannot be used to compare disability experiences in countries). Our interpretation is that the factor where disability prevalence shows high loadings can be explained by the methodology used which is independent of the social and economic status of a country (see Fig. 1).

In an attempt to identify a disability indicator in this data that could be comparable among countries, we also analyzed the distribution of the types of disability and the overall prevalence rates of single types of disability. The objective was to compare the percentage of very common types of disabilities among different countries and evaluate their correlation with the same social and economic variables. Assuming that the overall prevalence rates of

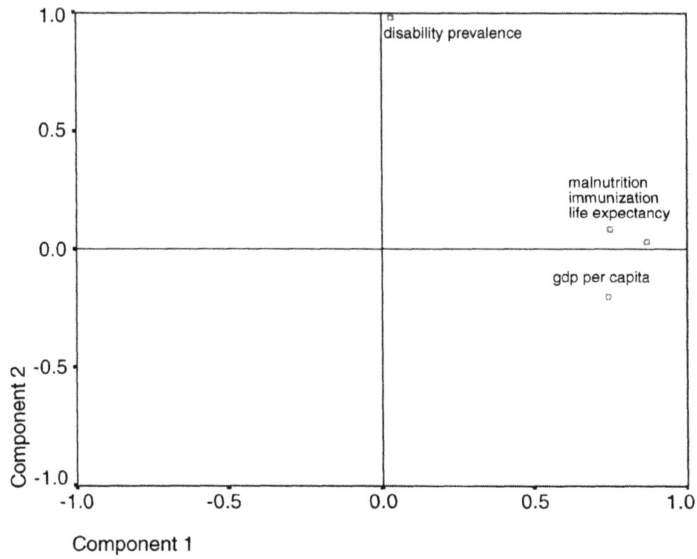

Fig. 1. Description of the Scores Obtained for Disability Prevalence Rates and Other Social and Economic Variables when Applying a Common Factor Analysis.

disability are not comparable because of different definitions and different methods used to identify the persons with disabilities, we wanted to see if the most visible types of impairments (such as blindness and deafness) were affected by this problem. The idea was to try to understand if there is a cultural pressure in developing countries to *always* report these impairments as disability regardless of the questions and approaches used to collect disability data. In order to understand if prevalence rates of selected types of impairments could be used to compare disability experiences among countries, we used the same analysis we undertook for total prevalence rates, looking at the statistical correlations between prevalence rates and social and economic indicators. We assumed that if we could observe a significant correlation between impairment rates and social and economic variables, the prevalence rates of these impairments could be used to compare disability experiences among countries.

Using preliminary data on types of disabilities in DISTAT-2 coded using the ICIDH (WHO, 1980), we analyzed three types of disabilities in countries where similar types of disabilities were collected: ocular impairments, aural impairments, and language impairments as percentage of total population and total number of persons with disabilities. We analyzed the linear correlation between these prevalence rates and the selected social-economic

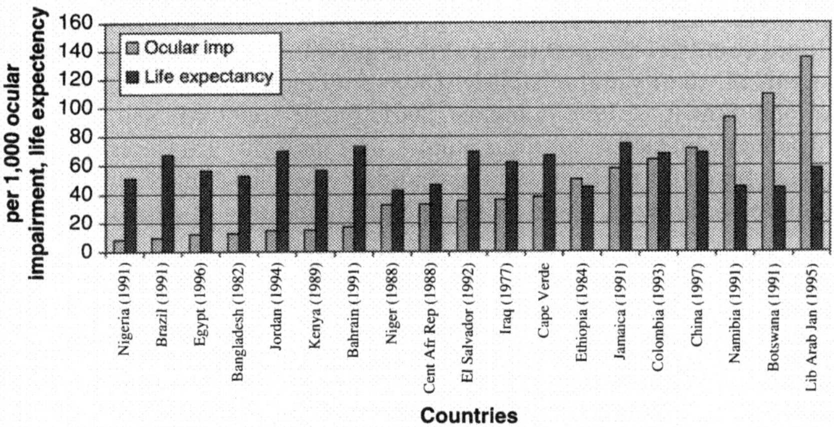

Fig. 2. Distribution of Prevalence of Ocular Impairment and Life Expectancy in Developing Countries.

indicators. Similarly from what we found for the total prevalence rate, there is no linear correlation between prevalence rates for each type of disability and the four social and economic variables. Fig. 2 shows an example of the different patterns of prevalence of ocular impairments and life expectancy.

The purpose of presenting the lack of relationship between disability prevalence and other indicators related to health, prevention, and economic prosperity is to show the problem related to the lack of uniform methodology used to collect disability prevalence rates and to argue that the methods used heavily affect the results and the interpretability of the data. The result of this analysis should not be interpreted as showing that disability is not related to the social and economic conditions of a country. On the contrary, we believe that disability is a crucial factor in understanding the social and health condition of different countries and regions of the world. The point that arises from the analysis is that disability data collected from countries still suffers from the lack of common methodologies and lack of common definitions. Unless this is taken into consideration in the analysis of the data, any comparison or interpretation can be mistaken.

HOW CAN THE MEASUREMENT OF DISABILITY BE IMPROVED?

There are some lessons that can be learned from the review of data collection methods used in developing countries on how measures of disability could be improved. There are also important results from studies carried out in developed countries to assess the quality of questions used to identify disability in terms of validity and reliability (Davis & Gligora, 2001; British Office for National Statistics, 1998; Langlois, 2001; Furrie, 1989; McNeil, 1993).

There is evidence in all these studies that disability measures can be improved. Based on the results of these studies, we believe that following issues should be considered when approaching the collection of data on disability:

- In many societies, there are *socio-cultural pressures* to underreport disability. It is important that in countries where disability is stigmatized, instruments to identify persons with disability be designed so that respondents do not perceive that they are being asked about the most stereotyped types of disabilities. It is also important that interviewers receive specialized training on *sensitivity*, with respect to asking questions on disability, *attitude*, in dealing with persons with disabilities, and *prejudice*, use of appropriate language, and inappropriate assumptions about a person's disability.
- The wording *of a question* has a great effect on the output of an instrument. Therefore, the language used should be clear, unambiguous, and simple. Negative terms should always be avoided. Testing of questions in Canada has shown, for example, that terms such as "long-term", "disability", and "handicaps" are viewed as extremely negative and tend to underreport disabilities (Langlois, 2001).
- The choice of *response categories* should be carefully evaluated to be sure that the respondent is not forced to associate him/herself with a stigma. In both Canada and Australia, use of scaled responses was found to improve the respondents' ability to report having disabilities. These findings are confirmed by other researchers who have argued that disability status is a complex phenomenon that involves multiple dimensions of health and severity. If the respondent cannot choose among these multiple dimensions, he/she is likely to misreport his/her disability status (Mathiowetz, 2000, 2001). It is argued that disability is not a "yes" or "no" phenomenon but rather a status that varies on a continuum in terms of intensity (mild disability) and time (cyclical disabilities). Alternatives such as *Yes sometimes*, *Yes often*, *No*[11] (Canada) or *None*, *A little*, *A lot*[12] (Australia) have proven to give better results.
- *Person*-based *questions* should be used instead of household-based questions if this does not compromise the overall interview time. The analysis of prevalence rates presented earlier showed that person-based questions are likely to identify a higher number of persons with disabilities than household-based questions. This finding is confirmed by Hess, Rothgeb,

Moore, Pascale, and Keeley (2001) where person-level questions were compared to household-level questions in a study carried out in the U.S. The data show that a person-level question identifies more people with functional limitations than a household-level question. However, the study also reports that household-level questions produce more reliable data than the person-level approach and in a shorter interview time.

- *Questions based on activity-limitations* and participation restriction should be considered instead of impairment-based questions in the design of general measures to identify persons with disabilities. An approach based on activity limitations includes a broader view of disability and it facilitates the collections of disability data by providing a more simple and neutral language (United Nations, 1998). It should be kept in mind that *disability is not an illness* (Chamie, 1995). Even when an impairment approach is used, diseases should not be included in the screening process and in the description of the types of disabilities.
- *The link between definitions, questions, and the description of types of disability* should be clear and consistent. Particular efforts should be made to translate the spirit of the definitions into the questions so that if an activity limitation approach is used for example in the definition, screening questions ask about limitations in activities and in the same line, the types of disabilities should include only activities.
- In designing census questions on disability special efforts should be made to address *special population groups* such as children, the elderly, and persons with psychological and cognitive impairments.[13]
- In applying the ICF framework, consideration should be given to the issue of maintaining *comparable time-series data*. In countries where data were collected in the past only in relation to the most severe types of disabilities, new questions oriented to broader definitions of disability should also capture these most severe types of disability. This would also address the need of users, particularly those at local level where the key population of interest for service planning is related to the most severe types of impairments (Davis & Gligora, 2001).[14]
- All the stakeholders, including persons with disabilities, should be involved in the activities in the planning process to collect, tabulate, and disseminate data on disability. A partnership between statisticians and the different data users needs to be established. The dialog should address the questions of "Why?", "Who?", and "What?" should be collected (United Nations, 2001a, b). Particularly where the resources are scarce and the available data collection methods can address only limited aspects of disability, both producers and users of disability statistics need to decide what the priorities are.

- Developing countries should be encouraged and supported to *test* new questions on disability based on the ICF. Questions that seem to have worked well in developed countries could be used in developing countries. However, the wording of these questions should be evaluated for their cultural sensitivity. In general, when new disability questions are developed, they should be evaluated for their validity and reliability in the context of the country before being used in national data collection activities.

There are other factors that may affect the reporting of disability in interviews, including cognition of different questions, use of proxy vs self-reporting,[15] question order, and the context in which the question is asked. Unfortunately there is little research on the impact of these characteristics on the quality of disability data particularly in developing countries. For this reason, one of the main conclusions of the United Nations Seminar on Measurement of Disability (held in New York from 4 to 6 June 2001) is the emphasis on the need for further research in these components of question design.[16]

TOWARD HARMONIZED APPROACHES IN THE MEASUREMENT OF DISABILITY

Although there are still many differences in the approaches used to collect disability data, many initiatives have been launched in the international arena with the objective of improving the harmonization of methodologies and the comparability of data. These initiatives include the approval of the ICF by WHO as the international standard to describe and categorize health and disability,[17] the development of sub-regional and international guidelines on measurement of disability, the establishment of the Washington Group on Disability Statistics and the organization of regional workshops on disability statistics by the United Nations Statistics Division (UNSD). The activities of the Washington Group are presented elsewhere in this volume.

UNSD is engaged in several efforts aimed at the improvement of methods of disability measurement and the development of common regional approaches to disability. In terms of international guidelines, a section on disability was included in the latest version of the *United Nations Principles and Recommendations for Population and Housing Censuses, Rev. 1* (United Nations, 1998). These recommendations give guidelines to countries on how to define the population with disabilities, develop the census question(s) to identify the population with disabilities, and tabulate the data on disability. The disability[18] concept as defined in the ICIDH (the predecessor of the ICF) is advocated to define the population with disabilities and it is suggested that questions on disability be framed in terms of activity limitations. Nine broad categories are suggested to describe the types of disabilities.[19] In preparation for the 2010 Population and Housing Census Decade, the United Nations is currently reviewing the Principles and Recommendations, and undoubtedly will update the section on disability to reflect, among other things, the application of the ICF in disability measurement. This will include use of the terminology of the ICF as well as its conceptualization of disability.

The forthcoming Recommendations for the 2010 Round of population and housing census by the United Nations Economic Commission for Europe will also include for the first time a section on disability with the purpose of harmonizing in the region the census collection of disability data under the framework of the ICF.

With the finalization of the *Guidelines and Principles for the Development of Disability Statistics* (United Nations, 2001b), the UNSD is organizing and conducting regional training workshops on disability statistics. The overall objective of these workshops is to strengthen national capabilities to produce, disseminate, and use data on disability for policy development and implementation. A specific objective of the workshops is to discuss the use of the ICF as the conceptual framework for collecting and classifying data and develop regional recommendations for disability measurement. At the workshops, participants from national statistical offices and data users from relevant government ministries are trained in how to identify disability data needs, and the use of the ICF concepts and definitions in the design of questions on disability and classification of the data. Conclusions of two of these workshops held in Africa and the Middle East are reported in United Nations (2001a, b, 2002).

CONCLUSIONS

Available information shows that there is a long history of collecting data on disability; for the most part, however, this has been done without the benefit of internationally agreed standards in terms of definitions, concepts or ways of collecting the information. The ICF provides a common framework for conceptualizing and defining disability. It offers a more comprehensive approach to disability measurement than has been traditionally done thereby increasing the relevance of the data to a wide set of users. The establishment of the Washington Group on Disability Statistics, in particular, and the overall work of the international organizations to strengthen the capacity of countries to collect data on disability and develop common improved methods, promise more comparable and more policy-relevant data on disability.

These international endeavors and also research and lessons learned from the past experience of countries provide valuable information on how to improve the collection of data on disability. However, much more needs to be done particularly in developing countries in terms of testing new methodologies and understanding the influence of different cultural factors on the reporting of disability.

NOTES

1. Further information on ICF is available on the ICF website: http://www.who.int/classification/icf.
2. DISTAT is a global database including statistics, indicators, and textual information from national data collected on disability issues.
3. These refer to crude disability rates.
4. Example of a household-based question is "Is there anybody in the household who is limited in his/her daily activities?" Example of a person-based question is "is…(name of the person) limited in his/her daily activities?"
5. The non-significant factors are not reported.
6. Most of the prevalence rates generated by developing countries are very low and are concentrated from 2% to –3%. 3% may not be considered "extremely high" in developed countries, but in developing countries these are not very common.
7. The analysis was done studying the ANOVA for categorical data.
8. Aruba (Census, 1991): "*Are you (or is she/she) handicapped?*"; Belize (Census, 1991): "*Does…suffer from any long-standing illness, disability or infirmity?*"; Bermuda (Census, 1991): "*Do you have a physical, mental or other health condition or limitation which has lasted for more than six months and which limits or prevents your participation in the activities of daily life e.g. work, recreation, mobility, schooling, etc.?*"; Saint Vincent and the Grenadines (Census, 1991): "*Does…suffer from any long-standing illness, disability or infirmity?*"
9. Information on this survey program can be found on the Internet at http://www.who.int/whs.
10. Vision, hearing, digestion, bodily excretion and continence, fertility, skin and disfigurement, breathing difficulty (dyspnea), pain and discomfort, affect, sleep, energy and vitality, understanding and interacting, communication, mobility and physical activity, dexterity and fine motor activity, self-care, interpersonal relationships, usual activities and roles (work, home, school, etc.), and social functioning (community activities).
11. These are response items related to the question: "*Does this person have any difficulty hearing, seeing, communicating, walking, climbing stairs, bending, learning or doing similar activities?*"
12. These are response items related to the question: "*How much difficulty does the person have in doing everyday activities such as eating, showering or dressing?*"

13. For example, the experience of the 1991 U.K. census shows that it is possible to improve the disability reporting of sup-population groups such as the elderly. A sentence was included at the end of the question: "*Include problems which are due to old age*" and the disability prevalence rate among elderly reported in the census was higher than the one reported in the survey (British Office for National Statistics, 1998).

14. The 2000 Census in Brazil is an example of this "mixed" approach. Questions related to very severe impairments and activity limitations were both included in the census questionnaire.

15. Some results obtained from the 1990 U.S. census and the Content Re-interview Survey reported by Nancy Mathiowetz (2000) shows that proxy respondents tend to report more activity limitations and more severe limitations than self-respondents. The impact of self and proxy reporting was also assessed in studies carried out by Tourangeau and Mathiowetz (2002) and Frey (2002) where no significant difference was observed on population estimates and reliability of measures. However, the impact of proxy or self-reporting is still uncertain in functional limi tations linked for example to mental and cognitive impairments.

16. More information on the meeting can be found at: http://www.un.org/Depts/unsd/disability/methods/index.html.

17. Further information on ICF is available on the ICF website: http://www.who.int/classification/icf.

18. In the context of health experience, a disability is any restriction or lack (resulting from an impairment) of ability to perform an activity in a manner or within the range considered normal for a human being (WHO, 1980).

19. (1) seeing difficulties (even with glasses, if worn); (2) hearing difficulties (even with hearing aid, if used); (3) speaking difficulties (talking); (4) moving/mobility difficulties (walking, climbing stairs, standing); (5) body movement difficulties (reaching, crouching, kneeling); (6) gripping/holding difficulties (using fingers to grip or handle objects); (7) learning difficulties (intellectual difficulties, retardation); (8) behavioral difficulties (psychological, emotional problems); (9) personal care difficulties (bathing, dressing, feeding).

20. Based on technical material provided by countries to the United Nations Statistics Division.

ACKNOWLEDGMENTS

We thank Jeremiah Banda, Erlinda Go, Nenad Kostanjsek, and Clare Menozzi for their valuable comments and suggestions on an earlier version of this paper.

REFERENCES

Altman, B. M. (2001). Definition of disability and their operationalization. *Research in Social Science and Disability*, *2*, 77–100.

British Office for National Statistics. (1998). Disability and care: Questions and needs considered. *Proceedings of a conference* held on 15 June, London.
Chamie, M. (1989). Survey design strategy for the study of disability. *World Health Statistics Quarterly*, *42*(3), 122–140.
Chamie, M. (1995). What does morbidity have to do with disability? *Disability and Rehabilitation*, *17*(7), 323–337.
Davis, E., & Gligora, C. (2001). Comparative analysis of censuses and surveys as instruments to collect data on disability – Australian experience. Paper presented by Ken Black at the United Nations seminar on measurement of disability, New York, 4–6 June.
Frey, W. (2002). Presentation made at the panel discussion: *The Social Security Administration's Disability Survey: Recommendations from the National Academy of Sciences' Committee.* American Statistical Association Meeting.
Furrie, A. D. (1989). *Comparison of the results from the 1989 census and the health and activity limitation survey for persons with disabilities residing in households.* Unpublished paper. 3 October.
Groce, N. E. (1999). Health beliefs and behavior towards individuals with disability cross-culturally. In: R. Leawitt (Ed.), *Cross-cultural rehabilitation: An international perspective.* Philadelphia: University of Pensylvania Press.
Hess, J., Rothgeb, J., Moore, J., Pascale, J., & Keeley, C. (2001). Measures of functional limitations: The effects of person-level vs. household-level questionnaire design. *Research in Social Science and Disability*, *2*, 145–166.
IOM. (2002). *The dynamics of disability, measuring and monitoring disability for social security programs.* U.S. Institute of Medicine and National Research Council, National Academy Press.
Jette, A. M., & Badley, E. (2000). Conceptual issues in the measurement of work disability. In: N. Mathiowetz & G. S. Wunderlich (Eds), *Survey measurement of work disability, summary of a workshop.* Washington, DC: National Academy Press.
Langlois, R. (2001). The development of a global disability indicator. Paper presented at the United Nations seminar on measurement of disability, New York, 4–6 June.
Mathiowetz, N. A. (2000). Methodological issues in the measurement of work disability. In: N. Mathiowetz & G. S. Wunderlich (Eds), *Survey measurement of work disability, summary of a workshop.* Washington, DC: National Academy Press.
Mathiowetz, N. A. (2001). Methodological issues in the measurement of persons with disabilities. *Research in Social Science and Disability*, *2*, 125–143.
Mbogoni, M. (2003). On the application of the ICIDH and ICF in developing countries: Evidence from the United Nations Disability Statistics Database (DISTAT). *Disability and Rehabilitation*, *25*(11–12), 644–658.
McNeil, J. (1993). Census bureau data in persons with disabilities: New results and old questions about validity and reliability. Paper presented at the 1993 annual meeting of the society for disability studies, Seattle, Washington, DC.
Pfeiffer, D. (2001). The conceptualization of disability. *Research in Social Science and Disability*, *2*, 29–52.
Tourangeau, R., & Mathiowetz, N. (2002). The measurement of persons with disabilities. Paper presented at the 2002 American statistical association meeting.
UNICEF. (1999). *An overview of young people living with disabilities: Their needs and their rights.* United Nations Children's Fund, September.

United Nations. (1990). *Disability statistics compendium.* United Nations publication, Sales No. E.90, XVII.17 (available on the Internet at: http://unstats.un.org/unsd/publication/SeriesY/SeriesY_4e.pdf).

United Nations. (1998). *Principles and recommendations for population and housing censuses, rev. 1.* United Nations Publication, Sales No. E.98, XVII.8 (available on the Internet at: http://unstats.un.org/unsd/publication/SeriesM/SeriesM_67rev1E.pdf).

United Nations. (2001a). *Report of the United Nations workshop on disability statistics for Africa.* United Nations Statistics Division (available on the Internet at: http://unstats.un.org/unsd/demographic/meetings/wshops/disab/Africa_rep.pdf).

United Nations. (2001b). *Guidelines and principles for the collection of disability statistics.* United Nations Publication, Sales No. E.01.XVII.15 (available on the Internet at: http://unstats.un.org/unsd/publication/SeriesY/SeriesY_10e.pdf).

United Nations. (2002). *Report of the meeting on disability measurement for ESCWA countries.* United Nations Statistics Division (available on the Internet at: http://unstats.un.org/unsd/demographic/meetings/wshops/disab/Cairo_rep.pdf).

WHO. (1980). *International classification of impairments, disabilities and handicaps.* Geneva, reprint 1993.

WHO. (2001). *International classification of functioning, disability and health.* Geneva.

ANNEX 1. : EXAMPLES OF DEFINITIONS USED IN CENSUSES[20]

Aruba, 1991

Handicapped persons are persons with a physical or a mental disorder. The handicap is formed by the limitations of the personal abilities due to the disorder.

Bahamas, 2000

A person with a disability is a person who is unable to ensure himself or herself, wholly or partly, the necessities of a normal individual and/or social life, as a result of a deficiency, either congenital, or not, in his or her physical or mental capabilities.

Cyprus, 1982

"Disabled person" means an individual whose prospects of securing and retaining suitable employment are substantially reduced as a result of physical or mental impairment.

Morocco, 1994

A disabled person is someone who is at a disadvantage to do something because of a deficiency or a physical or mental handicap. Deficiency is considered as a loss or anomaly of a structure or a psychological or anatomical function.

Nigeria, 1991

Disability has been defined as a restriction or lack (resulting from an impairment) of ability to perform an activity in the manner or within the range considered normal for a human being. Disability is characterized by excesses or deficiencies of customarily expected activity performance and behavior, and these may be temporary or permanent, reversible or irreversible, and progressive or regressive. Disabilities may arise as a direct consequence of impairment or as a response by the individual, particularly psychologically, to a physical, sensory, or other impairment. Disability represents objectification of an impairment, and as such if reflects disturbances at the level of the person. Therefore, disability is concerned with abilities, in the form of composite activities and behaviors, that are generally accepted as essential components of everyday life.

Pakistan, 1981

Disability refers to the physical or organic handicap of a person due to natural deformity or deficient functioning of any limb resulting from accident, disease, etc. It includes blind, deaf and dumb, crippled, mentally retarded, and insane.

Philippines, 1990

Disability refers to any restriction or lack (resulting from an impairment) of ability to perform an activity in the manner or within the range considered normal for a human being.

Poland, 1990

In the group disabled persons, legal and biological disabled persons are distinguished.

Legally disabled persons are defined as persons who possess a valid certificate of disability issued by the Commission on Disability and Employment stating the category of disability (i, ii, iii) whether they receive a disability pension or not.

Biologically disabled persons are defined as persons who at the time of the census stated that due to disability to perform everyday basic activities typical of a given age, such as: education, work, household duties – and for small children – playing. Two degrees of disability were distinguished: complete and severe disability. In both cases only long-term disability (over 6 months) caused by impairment of chronic diseases was considered.

Sri Lanka, 1981

Totally blind, totally deaf and/or dumb persons and persons with a disability in one or more legs or arms were regarded as physically disabled.

Uganda, 1991

A disability is defined as any condition that prevents a person from living normal social and working life.

West Bank and Gaza, 1996

A "restriction or lack (resulting from an impairment) of ability to perform an activity in the manner or within the range considered normal for a human being". It describes a functional limitation or activity restriction caused by impairment. Disabilities are description of disturbances in function at the level of the person. Examples of disabilities are difficulty in seeing, speaking, moving, climbing stairs, grasping, reaching, bathing, eating, and toiling.

Zambia, 2000

A person with a disability is defined as a person who is limited in the kind or amount of activities that he or she can do because of the ongoing difficulties due to a long-term physical condition, mental condition or health problem. Only disabilities lasting for more than six months should be included.

PRODUCTION, DISSEMINATION AND UTILIZATION OF DISABILITY STATISTICS IN UGANDA

Helen Namirembe-Nviiri

ABSTRACT

It is generally difficult for the government to come up with any meaningful programs for persons with disabilities (PWDs) unless statistics to that effect have been made available. Disability Statistics in Uganda is one of those areas of social statistics which has been growing at a slow pace in the past compared to other socioeconomic indicators, but now is an area of growing concern and picking up steadily. Censuses have remained the major data providers for disability statistics and the first of which was the 1991 census. The 2002 census similarly collected information on PWDs, and this information is to be widely disseminated at national and lower levels. Both censuses were conducted by the Uganda Bureau of Statistics (UBOS). UBOS has collected similar but a little more detailed information on disability using two household surveys.

However for effective program design, implementation and resource allocation for PWDs, a lot needs to be done in terms of harmonizing the concepts on disability with the International Classification of Functional Disability and Health (ICF). The power of the census results is that it provides data to the lowest administrative level. Conducting a fully

International Views on Disability Measures: Moving Toward Comparative Measurement
Research in Social Science and Disability, Volume 4, 89–109

ISSN: 1479-3547/doi:10.1016/S1479-3547(05)04007-8

fledged national survey for PWDs will provide adequate baseline data for meaningful purposes and priority issues for government and other users.

This report provides information on the various sources of disability data and how concepts are defined by each institution. It highlights the Uganda Bureau of Statistics, Ministry of Education and Sports (Annual School Census and the Department for Special Needs), Ministry of Gender, Labour and Social Development (Community-Based Rehabilitation Program) and the Ministry of Health as data collecting institutions. It is noted that each institution use different concepts and methodology for data collection. Engaging both users and producers in the disability data production process, encouraging regular dialogue and establishing collaborative arrangements with local and international research institutions are avenues for utilizing the scarce resources for the development of disability statistics. The focus and direction of the development of disability statistics in Uganda calls for a sustained system of monitoring intervention that government and other development partners have to put in place.

The issues raised in this report will facilitate the process of harmonisation of concepts and definitions used while collecting disability data. It is noted that except for the Community-Based Rehabilitation Information pilot system under the Ministry of Gender, Labour and Social Development, there is little or no use at all of the ICF. The pilot system is ongoing and is expected to expand to other districts. It is hoped that this will enrich the process of harmonizing concepts with the Integrated Community-Based Rehabilitation Information System to provide meaningful results. The process of coordination is hereby called for.

BACKGROUND

Various nations have been recognizing the rehabilitation needs and civil rights of people with disability (PWDs) as well as the effects of impairment and disability on national indicators of health, education and economic prosperity. This has created dire need for information for policy makers and program managers in all these key areas. Information needs range from basic need of counts of the number of PWDs, their education levels, where they are residing, etc, to more complex issues like making comparisons on the quality of life for those persons with disabilities as compared to those persons without disabilities.

In Uganda, the Governments commitment towards persons with disabilities dates back to shortly after independence in 1965 when a data collection exercise for persons with disabilities was commissioned. The study revealed that about 10 per cent of the country's population were disabled and that approximately 6,000 persons were becoming disabled annually. In the light of this problem the Government, with International Labour Organization (ILO) support, developed a National Vocational Rehabilitation Scheme to provide persons with disabilities, social and economic independence.

Over the last few years, there has been increased awareness about disability and the corresponding inclusion of service provision for the persons with disabilities in Uganda. There are different sectors that undertake programs for PWDs. Throughout the implementation of their programs, they undertake data gathering processes as measures to facilitate implementation of their programs. The collection of these data and production of data on disability is therefore an issue of growing concern.

This paper reviews the different institutions that generate data on disability in Uganda. It highlights the objective of collecting the data, the type of questions used and any accompanying guideline instructions. The methods used to disseminate the information are also highlighted. These institutions include;

- Uganda Bureau of Statistics
- Ministry of Gender, Labour and Social Development
- Ministry of Health
- Ministry of Education and Sports and
- Various Non-Governmental Organizations (NGOs) like the Uganda National Society for Disabled Children, etc.

Uganda Bureau of Statistics (UBOS)

The UBOS was established in 1998 under the Statistics Act. Prior to its establishment, the former Statistics Department had been involved in conducting Censuses and Household Surveys. In addition, in 1991 the former Statistics Department conducted a nationwide population and housing census, which has been the major source of data on disability at the national, district and lower levels.

Disability Data from the 1991 Population and Housing Census

The 1991 Population and Housing Census was conducted after a period of 21 years without census data.[1] Because of this data gap, there was a lot of pressure to include a great variety of questions on the census questionnaire.

The final version of the questionnaire was a compromise between the high demand for data and the high cost of data collection.

The 1991 census was conducted in a "census-cum-sample" format. Two questionnaires (short and long) were used. The long questionnaire was administered to all households in urban areas and in a 10 per cent sample of the rural areas, while the short questionnaire was administered to the rest of the population. In effect, the exercise was a complete count of the population with a simultaneous sample survey of some individual and household characteristics.

Questions on Disability

The section of Rehabilitation under the Department of Community Development in the Ministry of Local Government (among others) requested the Statistics Department to collect information on disability during the 1991 census. The prime objective of collecting these data was to "*to determine (the) disabled population by age, sex, disability condition and causes*". This information to be collected included the following:

Questions on Disability (as proposed by Ministry of Local Government)

Sex Male Female

Nature of Disability	**Cause of Disability**
Blind	Born with
Mentally ill	Disease
Mentally retarded	Accident
Deaf and Dumb	Inflicted injury
Polio	Others
Amputee	
Leprosy	**Conditions**
Epilepsy	Severe
Hunchback	Moderate
Others N.E.S	Slight

However, the pilot census did not collect any information on disability. The main census enumeration included two questions on disability of the three that had been proposed, on the long questionnaire. There were no questions on disability on the short questionnaire. The questions and the corresponding Enumerators' Instructions are as given below.

Disability Questions

Is Anyone Who Was In The Household On The Census Night Disabled?
Yes Or No
If Yes, Write: Person Number

Nature of Disability: blind, mentally ill, deaf and dumb, polio, amputee, leprosy, cripple, lame, epilepsy, mentally retarded, other (specify).

Cause of Disability: born, disease, accident, inflicted injury etc

Enumerator's Instruction

DISABILITY
175 "*Is anyone who was in the household on the census night disabled?*"

Nature of Disability

176 By "disabled" we mean any condition which prevents a person from living a normal, social and working life.

177 There are many disabilities and conditions which may prevent a person from living a normal life. And they may be difficult to describe accurately. But most people have a good idea of what amounts to disability, and for census purposes we have to rely on your judgement and that of the household and person concerned.

178 There are clear cases of disability such as having lost a leg, or being so crippled by polio that one cannot walk normally, or being mad. There are many cases where it is not so easy. In such cases, common sense must be your guide. If the condition is not so serious as to prevent a person from living a full life and being able to provide for him or herself, it should not be counted as a disability.

179 If a person has lost an arm, he or she is disabled. A person who has lost the tip of a finger in an accident would not normally be considered disabled. In the same way a person whose sight is impaired but who wears glasses and can live and work normally while doing so is not disabled for purposes of the census. For census purposes old age is not a disability.

180 If there is anyone in the household who is disabled or whom you and others think of as disabled, write the person number and describe the nature of the disability as best you can in a few words. It is important that you write the person number because we need to know the sex, age and other particulars of the person concerned.

Cause of Disability

181 People may be born with a disability. They may be disabled as a result of illness or because of an injury received by accident or because of an injury inflicted on them by others. Describe the cause as best you can.

Although the request was made to collect information on the "condition" of disability, this was excluded partly because the classifications were very subjective (i.e. severe, moderate and not severe). It would thus be difficult to obtain standard information from the *respondents*. The following codes were adopted for processing the data:

Nature of Disability	Cause of Disability
1. Blind	1. Born
2. Deaf/Dumb	2. Disease
3. Amputee	3. Accident
4. Leper	4. War Injury
5. Epileptic	5. All Others
6. Cripple/Lame	6. Not Reported
7. Mentally Retarded	
8. Others N.E.S.	
9. Not Reported	

The census realized a total of 190,435 disabled persons among the household population of Uganda (implying a disability rate of 1.1 per cent). This is lower than what was presumed to be the general level of disability by WHO of 10 per cent.

Data Quality. The national level analysis, resulted in reservations about the quality of the data. There was concern about the level of coverage for several reasons. This is clearly stated in the census report. The relevant text is reproduced below.

The definition used by the census is not as detailed as that used by other studies such as the World Health Organisation (WHO). In addition, census enumerators were not well trained in the identification of disability. Further, such information was not collected from institutional populations. This hence excluded the disabled in institutions. This exclusion may have had a significant consequence on the volume of the disabled population. Consequently, the information collected has an under enumeration of the disabled, and it shows the minimum level of disability in the country.

Source: The 1991 Population and Housing Census, Analytical Report, Volume II, Page 125.

However, despite the possible under enumeration mentioned above, it was believed that the data were useful as regards patterns (i.e. sex, age type of disability, by region/district, etc) and varieties of the disabled, and these formed the basis of the analysis.

Topics used in analysis of Disability Data

Sex Composition of Disabled Population
Age Composition of Disabled Population
Disabled Population by Regions/Districts

Because of the limitation already mentioned above and the fact that the actual number of disabled persons identified was low, no other tabulations or analysis of disability data by additional characteristics were done.

In essence, the analysis carried out all the possible tabulations of the disability data from the census. This unfortunately did not satisfy the data needs in respect of disability. This is more so given the fact that no individual characteristics of the disabled persons other than age, sex and spatial distribution were studied.

The resulting data are published in the 1991 Census Publications (i.e. Analytical Report, Volume II, Main Release, District Summary Reports). At present, UBOS established a web site (http://www.ubos.org) where some of the census data are disseminated.

THE 2002 POPULATION AND HOUSING CENSUS

Preparatory work for the 2002 Population and Housing Census included a pre-test and a Pilot Census. The proposed questionnaire was pre-tested in July 2001 and the Pilot Census took place in September 2001. This time the census was "piggy backing" an agricultural module to generate a sampling frame for future Agricultural Censuses.

Unlike the previous census where two questionnaires (short and long) were administered, one questionnaire (long) was administered to every household. The questionnaire included 3 (three) questions on Disability as follows:

13. DISABILITY: Does (NAME) have any difficulty in moving, seeing, hearing, speaking or learning which has lasted or is expected to last 6 months or more?
(If NO write 10 & skip to P.16) If YES, write codes at most 2 major difficulties) Types of disability are identified in terms of impairments and chronic conditions

14. CAUSE OF DISABILITY: What caused this difficulty? Causes of disability are identified by the source of the problem either from disease or as the result of birth defects, or some kinds of injury.
(Write the code for cause for each corresponding difficulty.)

15. REHABILITATION/ASSISTANCE OF DISABILITY: What measures are being used by (NAME) to minimise on the impact of the difficulty?

The above questions were asked to each member of the household and it took care of multiple disability, i.e. a maximum of two types of disabilities were recorded for each person.

The codes provided in the questionnaire for questions 13,14 and 15 are given as follows:

Code	**Type of Disability (P13)**	**Cause of Disability (P14)**	**Rehabilitation of Disability (P15)**
10.	None	10. Congenital (born with a disability)	10. None
11.	Limited use of legs	11. Disease /illness	11. Surgical Operation

12.	Loss of leg(s)	12. Transport accident	12. Medication
13.	Limited use of arms	13. Occupational Injury	13. Assistive Devices
14.	Loss of arm(s)	14. Other Accident	14. Special Education (mentally retarded)
15.	Serious problem with back spine	15. War	15. Braille Training
16.	Hearing difficulty	16. Natural ageing process	16. Skills Training (vocational)
17.	Unable to hear (Deafness)	17. Other causes (specify)	17. Sign language training
18.	Sight difficulty		18. Counseling
19.	Blindness		19. Others (specify)
20.	Speech impairment		
21.	Unable to speak (mute)		
22.	Mental retardation		
23.	Mental illness (strange behaviour)		
24.	Epileptic		
25.	Rheumatism		
26.	Others (specify)		

An accompanying manual of instruction was prepared and the instructions on how to fill the above questions are given as follows:

Disability

1. A person with a disability is defined as the one who is limited in the kind of or amount of activities that he or she can do, because of ongoing difficulty(ies) due to a long-term physical condition or health problem that has lasted **6 months or more**. This includes all those difficulties that are expected to last more than 6 months.
2. Note that a person can have a fractured arm or leg due to a road accident and is expected to heal within 3 months. For purposes of the census, you should not record this person to have a difficulty since the difficulty is expected to last for a shorter period.
3. There are some clear cases of disability such as having lost a leg, or being crippled by polio that one cannot walk normally, or being

mad. However, there are also many cases where it is not so clear. In such cases, common sense must be your guide. If the respondent indicates that the condition is not so serious as to prevent a person from living a full life, it should not be counted as a disability.

4. If a person has lost an arm, he or she is disabled. A person who has lost the tip of a finger in an accident should not be considered as disabled. In the same way, a person whose sight is impaired but can live and work normally by wearing glasses while doing so is not disabled for purposes of the census.
   Question P13: **Disability**
   Ask, "Does (NAME) have any difficulty in moving, seeing, hearing, speaking difficulty, mental or learning difficulty, which has lasted or is expected to last 6 months or more?"
5. If the respondent declares anyone in the household as disabled, use the codes in the questionnaire and describe the nature of the disability as best as you can. Some persons with disabilities have more than one type of disability. In this case you are required to take the two major forms of disability and assign the appropriate codes in the space provided. Note that the column for each person takes care of two types of disabilities.
6. It is quite common for persons in the household to hide information about disabilities of their kins, especially the children. Ensure that you attempt to see and probe to obtain the truth.
7. Examples of such categories of persons include, those who have:

Seeing Difficulties: An individual could have a sight problem if he/she cannot see clearly objects that are close to him/her or is unable to figure out objects, which are at a distance. Note that if one wears glasses and ceases to have a problem with sight, then he/she does not qualify to be recorded as having any seeing difficulties. A separate code for "Blindness" is provided for persons who cannot see at all. If a person has lost one eye, this does not automatically imply that he has a sight problem. Ask the respondent to find out if he/she has a sight difficulty and assign the appropriate code.

Hearing Difficulties: This includes persons those who have difficulty in hearing i.e. not following a conversation in a normal voice even with use of a hearing aid. In case an individual has a hearing aid and is able to follow a conversation in a normal voice, then he/she does not have a hearing difficulty. A separate code for unable to hear (deaf) is included for those who cannot hear at all.

Speech Impairment: Includes persons with problems of speech, even though they are able to hear. Those who are not able to speak at all are categorised as "Mute".

Mental Illness (Strange Behaviour): This is characterised by strange behaviours and the most common description is mad.

Learning Difficulty/Mental Retardation: This includes persons with learning difficulties in or out of school and persons mentally less developed than their age mates. They can be adults or children.

Epilepsy: This is a condition where a person has episodes of loss or change of consciousness that may last from a few seconds to over an hour. The loss of consciousness is sometimes accompanied by movement of body parts. The loss of consciousness is also called fit. Epilepsy fits are NOT accompanied by fever.

Rheumatism: This is of when the joints of a body are swollen, hot and painful. It is often accompanied by limited movement of the joint.

Question P14: **Cause of Disability**

Ask, "What caused this difficulty?"

8. Causes of disability are important because they provide the health and medical explanation of the disability. This information is useful in providing preventive measures against the disability. For example, a person may have difficulty in walking because he/she suffered from leprosy or polio. Similarly, a person with strange behaviour or mental retardation may have suffered from a long illness, which affected the brain.
9. Sometimes people may be born with a disability. They may be disabled as a result of an illness or because of an injury caused by an accident or because of an injury inflicted on them by others. Record the code of the cause for each corresponding type of disability recorded in P13.

Question P15: **Rehabilitation/Assistance of Disability**

Ask, "What measures are being taken by (NAME) to minimise the impact of the difficulty?"

10. Rehabilitation is a process with a target within a time frame aimed at enabling a person with a disability to reach a certain mental, physical and/ or social functional level, thus providing the skills/ tools to change his/her own life.

11. Record the rehabilitation undertaken for each measure corresponding to each nature of disability. Below are a few guidelines:
    - **Special Education:** Giving the person special types of education for the mentally retarded.
    - **Medical Rehabilitation:** This is the use of surgery, or doing special exercises like physiotherapy and medication etc.
    - **Assistive Devices:** Such as clutches, walking sticks, wheel chairs, calipers, artificial limbs, hearing aids etc.
    - **Vocational Rehabilitation:** Provides equipment and services to people with disabilities to improve their ability to work or to live not as dependants. For example, provision of training on how to earn a living. Such training includes, shoe making, weaving, etc.

According to the 2002 Census Main Report, the disability rate was 4 per cent (actually 3.5 per cent), compared to 3.3 per cent using the international definition. The prevalence rate in 2002 was higher than 1.1 per cent obtained for the 1991 census. The percentage increase is partly attributed to improvements in the method of data collection used in the 2002 census.[2]

Other Household Surveys with Disability Modules

UBOS is conducting the following two household surveys (i) the 2004 Northern Uganda Baseline Survey covering 18 districts in Northern Uganda for the Northern Uganda Social Action Fund Program, and (ii) the 2005/2006 Uganda National Household Survey (UNHS III). Both surveys are funded by the World Bank. The modules for each survey are slightly different but the manual is the same. The 2005/2006 questions are a subset of the 2004 Northern Uganda Survey.

MINISTRY OF GENDER, LABOUR AND SOCIAL DEVELOPMENT (MGLSD)

The MGLSD, through the Department of Disability and Elderly, is mandated by the Government of Uganda, to play an integral role in the design and implementation of the Community-Based Rehabilitation Program (CBR) and Vocational Rehabilitation in the country for PWDs. The Government of Uganda adopted the CBR as an appropriate service strategy to reach more PWDs in 1992.

The program is operational in 26 districts in the country. Within each district, a number of subcounties are covered annually by the CBR program.

The project has the following components:

- Identifying PWD and assessing their needs
- Making home visits and counseling
- Making appropriate referrals to services
- Mobilization of PWDs to form groups
- Promoting disabled person roles in the community through cultural activities
- Developing appropriate appliances for PWDs
- Training of CBR workers

In each subcounty, PWDs are identified and registered by the community though sensitization meetings. The local council chiefs, local council executives or the PWDs themselves can act as principal notifiers to the Community Development Assistants (CDAs), the CDAs in return may take the Doctor to the community to treat the PWDs from the community. The CDA work hand in hand with the Special Needs Education Coordinator.

The type of data collected includes:
Number of persons with disabilities by type of disability, age sex and cause of disability and by District

Objectives of data collection are for planning purposes like improving service delivery and to provide proper intervention guidelines for program implementation. The PWDs are identified by the community and the CDA takes a profile of each PWD by filing the Community-Based Rehabilitation Management Information System questionnaire. This information is sent to the District Rehabilitation Centre where it is captured and analysed.

The Pilot Community-Based Rehabilitation Information System

The Ministry is currently developing a Data Management Information System on disability statistics in the program districts. The pilot exercise program started in one District of Tororo, and will finally be expanded to cover other districts.

Purpose

(i) To establish an adequate capacity of supervision, monitoring and reporting for the CBR program.
(ii) To develop information systems that not only satisfy the specified needs but can also adapt to the conditions in the districts as regards compilation and processing of data.

A PWD is defined as one who has difficulties/restrictions in performing daily activities leading to failure to participate like other people. If a person experiences difficulty in one or more of the following areas, they can be considered to have a disability; seeing, hearing, speaking (using language or conveying messages), moving around or using body parts, learning, fits, has strange behaviour, loss of skin feeling, and others not mentioned here.

The following forms are used to generate the data on PWD:

1. Identification, registration and baseline information forms – collect individual information in a community using the types of disabilities mentioned above (seeing, hearing, speaking,..., strange behaviour, etc). It has no option for multiple disabilities. The information is summarized from lower levels up to District level
2. Assessment, follow up and referral forms – these have options for multiple disabilities and the PWD is assessed in the community where he/she lives on different days. Information is detailed and can be linked to the ICF.
3. Supervision and monitoring guidelines
4. Reporting guidelines

The process of assessing the PWD is as follows:
In assessing abilities and inabilities, the Community Workers (Health Special Needs Education Coordinators, Community Development Assistants, Community Bases Rehabilitation Officers) take care and observe the PWD carrying out specific activities before recording. The assessment includes the areas of self-care, speaking and conveying messages, learning, mobility, pain, strange behaviour, gainful occupation, attitude, fits and loss of feeling (skin sensation).

Severity of disability is recorded as mild, moderate or severe. This is from the community workers' point of view. The duration and cause of disability is also recorded. It also takes care of all domains of well-being (i.e. seeing, speaking, education, employment, etc.).

Observation checklist is also filled because it is important to give attention to the environment since rehabilitation depends on the home and community environment. The following issues are included for observation:

- Home environment (in terms of cleanliness, behaviour)
- Accessibility (in terms of space, number of people in the home, facilities, distance to social services, terrain of the place)
- Nutritional practices (whether the family has adequate food supplies)
- Hygiene of PWD
- Waste disposal
- Source of water
- Cultural beliefs/practices related to PWD

In general, there is a typology of questions listed below that addresses the above issues (severity, domain, duration and etiology):

- Identification of a disability
- Indication of limitation in activities
- Indication of difficulty
- Combination questions

Question Characteristics

All questions in the assessment form have a scale that ranges from 1 to 4. For example, a person moving independently will score 1, with difficulty-2, with greater difficulty-3, with no movements at all-4. In some instances where it is not applicable the score is X; for example, a 2-month-old child is not expected to walk.

At the end of each section, there is a total score and there is a summary table for total scores, that are recorded for each aspect of development. Reduction in total score indicates progress.

This assessment is done after 3 to 4 months to detect progress and to discharge clients from specific rehabilitation program, i.e. it can be partial or complete discharge.

Body functions	**Availability in assessment form**
Chapter 1: Mental functions	Yes
Chapter 2: Sensory functions and pain	Yes
Chapter 3: Voice and speech functions	Yes
Chapter 4: Functions of the cardiovascular, haematological, immunological and respiratory	No

Chapter 5: Functions of the digestive, metabolic and endocrine systems	No
Chapter 6: Genitourinary and reproductive functions	No
Chapter 7: Neuromusculoskeletal and movement-related functions	No
Chapter 8: Functions of the skin and related structures	Yes
Body Structures	Nil
Activity and Participation	No
Chapter 1: Learning and applying knowledge	Yes
Chapter 2: General tasks and demands	Yes
Chapter 3: Communication	Yes
Chapter 4: Mobility	Yes
Chapter 5: Self-care	Yes
Chapter 6: Domestic life	Yes
Chapter 7: Interpersonal interactions and relationships	
Chapter 8: Major life areas	Yes
Chapter 9: Community, social and civic life	Yes
Environment Factors	No
Chapter 1: Products and technology	No
Chapter 2: Natural environment and man-made changes to environment	Yes
Chapter 3: Support and relationships	Yes
Chapter 4: Attitudes	Yes
Chapter 5: Services, systems and policies	No

Mapping these data to ICF

In order to understand this approach of measuring disability and how the questions relate to international measures, this disability collection method has been mapped to the ICF. Some of the chapters have not been touched at all; in others at least one of the components is touched. The constructs/qualifier of "body structures" is not mentioned at all, as shown in the table.

MINISTRY OF EDUCATION AND SPORTS (MOES)

The MOES has two departments that are involved in generating statistics on disability, namely, the Department for Special Education Needs and the

Planning Department. The Planning Department is responsible for the collection and analysis of data from all government and non-government institutions in the country. The department for Special Education Needs in the same Ministry only focuses on pupils/students with disabilities.

Planning Department

The planning department of the MOES conducts annual school censuses throughout the country. The objective of collecting these data is basically for planning purposes, for instance, to guide the Ministry on the number of teachers with special needs and the number of scholastic materials for each district that are required.

Questionnaires for the annual school census are designed and the data collection process involves the following stages:

(i) Designing the questionnaire and accompanying manual of instructions for pre-testing. The pre-test is conducted in a few selected districts by a team of staff from headquarters. Thereafter comments from the field visits are incorporated to finalize the questionnaire publication.
(ii) A training is conducted for trainers, who include all District Education Officers, District Inspectors of School and Chief Administrative Officers is conducted.
(iii) District training workshops for School Head teachers and county Education officers are conducted thereafter.

Type of Data Collected

The school census questionnaire had different sections, and the section for pupils with disabilities is indicated as follows:

C.5. Pupils with Special Learning Needs by Class and Gender

	P1		P2		P3		P4		P5		P6		P7		**Total**	
	M	F	M	F	M	F	M	F	M	F	M	F	M	F	M	F
Mentally retarted																
Visually impaired																
Hearing impaired																
Physically impaired																
Autism																
Multiple handicaps (e.g. deaf and blind)																

The instructions for completion of the above section are given as follows:

> **C.5. Pupils with Special Learning Needs by Class and Gender** – for each grade write the number of pupils with special learning needs who may require specially trained teachers and/or teaching materials. To the right of the row (line) that lists the MAIN special learning need, write the total number of children by class and Gender in the appropriate cell. For example, if a child possesses more than one impairment, he/she should be included in the "Multiple Handicaps" category. Make sure that the separate figures for Males and Females agrees with the Total. The total for this item should **be less than, or at most, equal to** the total number of pupils enrolled as indicated on C.1. *(Note: Autism refers to that pupil or those pupils who for any reason have a failure to develop social abilities, language and other communication skills to the usual level, together with a severe limitation on the number of person's or persons' activities and interests).*

The data are published and disseminated in the Education Statistics Abstract.

The Special Needs Education (SNE)/Educational Assessment and Resource Services (EARS) Program.

This is a District program, that was established in 1992 between the governments of Uganda and Denmark. The program that was originally funded by Danida has been integrated in the MOES as a Department for Special Education and Carrier Guidance and has centres in each district throughout the country.

Initially the program covered children less than 18 years who are in school. The scope of this program has been broadened to cover all pupils and students attending formal education, i.e. those attending primary, secondary and university levels of education. It excludes those attending tertiary institutions (e.g. like Teacher Training Institutions, Technical Schools, etc).

The objective of the Special Needs Education program is to provide a comprehensive program of assistance to learners in both primary and secondary schools. The program aims at providing the needed support to these learners, parents, teachers and service providers.

A comprehensive approach to Special Needs Education includes the following activities:

- Early identification of learners with Special Education Needs
- Creation of awareness about learners with barriers to learning and development

- Prevention of conditions that can give difficulties or other barriers to learning and development
- Early interventions and subsequent inclusion of learners with SNE into mainstream
- Training parents, teachers, local administrator and others in meeting the SNE of these learners
- Developing and promoting appropriate assessment tools and education materials for learners with SNE
- Providing training, which can ensure that all teachers in primary schools receive basic education and knowledge on SNE
- Working in close co-operation with the other service providers to an efficient, complete range of services to learners with SNE
- Working alongside Non-Government Organizations, in particular the NUDIPU.

Types of Data Collected and Objectives of Collecting Data

The objectives of collecting these data are to assist and organize policies regarding formal education of PWDs attending Primary to University levels of education.

The data collection procedures involve Assistant Inspectors of schools in charge of special education who are located at each sub-county in the programme districts. These are assisted by Special Needs Education Co-ordinators (SNECOs), who are located at community level. Each SNECO is in charge of a catchment area of about 10–15 schools.

The questionnaires are designed at headquarters and sent to each District for the SNECOs to fill. The type of data collected by SNE/EARS includes the following:

1. District
2. Name, Address of SNECO?
3. State your Education in SNE?
4. Have you enrolled for a UNISE distance course in SNE?
5. How many teachers are enrolled in the individual schools for a UNISE distance-learning course?
6. How many schools are there in your cluster (by public, private)?
7. Does the school have a teacher in charge of SNE?
8. Number of children with disabilities by class and sex

Data Analysis and Dissemination

The data are collected and returned to the centre where it is analysed and published in annual reports. The following are some of the tables that are used in the analysis:

a) Number of children with special needs by class, sex, district and by type of disability
b) Type of special school by district
c) Number of trained teachers in SNE by level of training and by district
d) Number of teachers with SNE by type of SNE by district

The data are presented in user tables that serve as input data for planning purposes and program implementation. The data are also published in annual reports.

MINISTRY OF HEALTH (MOH)

A number of hospitals prepare annual reports to the Ministry of Health. These reports are based on the total number of inpatient admissions, which are classified by the number of diagnoses made, most of which are not related to disability. The records are used to generate data for planning purposes. The same data are used to analyse those diagnoses that are most related to disability. The data are analysed by number of cases admitted (in-patient cases) and number of morbidity cases. Plans are underway to include data on disability as part of the Health Management Information System (HMIS).

OTHER ORGANIZATIONS/NGOs

There are other organizations that are involved in collecting and compiling statistics on disability in Uganda. These include the following:

Uganda society for disabled children; a program which is operational in nine Districts. This is an NGO that supports Community-Based Rehabilitation Programs. The CBR programs involve home-based rehabilitation, outreach clinics and referrals to other services. They prepare annual reports to USDC Kampala headquarters.

The OURS Program is based in Mbarara District at the East Ankole Diocese. The CBR program identifies and refers people with disabilities in six subcounties through home-based programs.

CONCLUSION

It is very clear that the only source of nationwide data on disability statistics in Uganda is from censuses. It is also clear that the census cannot include comprehensive information on disability statistics that is required by all key stakeholders for planning and improvement of service delivery for PWDs. Yet the information collected by individual stakeholders can only serve their specific needs as opposed to those of the entire nation. In view of this, there is need to conduct more comprehensive surveys on disability to cover all areas that are required by the key stakeholders of disability statistics in Uganda. Second it is clear that the concept of the use of the ICF is new in Uganda like in many African countries. It is therefore important that the use of the ICF in the collection of disability statistics should be expanded as soon as possible. This will improve the comparability of data across countries.

NOTES

1. The 1980 population census lost most of its questionnaires before being processed.
2. Uganda Bureau of Statistics (UBOS). "The 2002 Uganda Population and Housing Census – Main Report", March 2005, Kampala, Uganda.

PARADIGMS LOST: THE CHANGING FACE OF DISABILITY IN RESEARCH

Mitchell E. Loeb and Arne H. Eide

ABSTRACT

Concepts of disability have evolved over the past few decades. The focus of attention has shifted from disability as a state, a consequence of disease, to disability being included as just one of many components of health. This has been realised in part through the implementation of the International Classification of Functioning, Disability and Health (ICF). Despite these developments and increased focus in recent years, reliable disability data, particularly from low-income countries, are lacking. We present an innovative approach to measuring disability in a population that is based on some conceptual elements of the ICF, namely activity limitations and participation restrictions. The results are derived from studies on the living conditions among people with disabilities in Namibia, Zimbabwe and Malawi conducted between 2001 and 2004. From the data analysis perspective, the research challenge lies in a shift in the dependent variable from a dichotomous outcome measure (disability as a state: disabled, not disabled) to a continuous measure of activity limitations and participation restrictions – mirroring the range of disability we see in society. These measures of activity limitations and participation restrictions must however not be interpreted in isolation, but as integral to the

International Views on Disability Measures: Moving Toward Comparative Measurement
Research in Social Science and Disability, Volume 4, 111–129

ISSN: 1479-3547/doi:10.1016/S1479-3547(05)04008-X

environment, society and culture from which they are derived. This will require an expanded view of disability data and effect substantially greater measurement challenges.

INTRODUCTION

In November of 2001 the World Health Organisation (WHO) launched the International Classification of Functioning, Disability and Health (ICF) marking the culmination of a task that spanned over two decades. The act of agreeing upon an internationally approved and standardised approach to classifying disability has underscored a major shift in the frame of reference with respect to disability – a paradigm shift that marked the transition from regarding disability as a "consequence of disease" to incorporating it within a broader "components of health" spectrum. From being a static label defining impairment, disability is understood as a process or an experience defining both activity limitations and participation restrictions and integral to the environment in which one lives.

In epidemiological research the approach to a problem is often delineated by the definition of the "case" we wish to describe or study. When the "case" in question is "disability" and it, in turn, is so closely linked to morbidity (physical or psychological limitation) we find ourselves bound to that particular paradigm. The tools at our disposal are determinants of morbidity; for example, measures of incidence and prevalence. Research has thus often focused, in part, on counting who is disabled in a population basically by asking the question: "What is wrong with you?"

By placing disability within a "components of health" spectrum, however, the focus of our attention shifts from one's static condition to a more process-oriented holistic view and the methodology we choose can be guided by answering the question: "What do you need to become a fully active and integrated member of your society?"

In that respect, the ICF has chosen to approach disability by focussing on how people live with their health condition. Rather than merely classifying or grouping individuals according to their physical, mental or psychological impairment, the ICF classifies health and health-related domains that describe body functions and structures as well as activities and participation. The domains are classified from body, individual and societal perspectives. Since an individual's functioning and disability are not independent from each other, the ICF also takes environmental factors into consideration (WHO, 2001a).

In a research setting, the two divergent disability paradigms outlined above beg different means of measurement that will necessarily provide different results. Regardless of the path we choose, however, we are obliged to define the population of interest: "Who is disabled?"

According to World Programme of Action Concerning Disabled Persons (UN, 1982), the UN estimated that in most countries at least 10% of the population is disabled by a physical, mental or sensory impairment. The large majority of disabled people live in developing or low-income countries,[1] very often living without optimal technical, medical or social support that could have improved their level of living conditions considerably. Disabled people are often marginalised and belong to the poorest segments of society (UN, 1982).

Using the WHO's benchmark of 10%, there would be about 650 million persons with disabilities worldwide today.

Two major problems face those interested in studying or determining the extent of disability in a population. One is deciding upon an acceptable definition for disability. There is no commonly accepted definition, no "neutral language" (Altman, 2001) and no standard test for disability that is constant from one population or society to another. Furthermore, if we presume to assess disability in its context, the definition is further complicated by the fact that there does not exist a standard or uniform environment in which disability (or the environmentally adjusted ability of an individual) may be measured that is common, or commonly understood among global societies. It is beyond the scope of this paper to review the literature concerning the problem surrounding a definition of disability, though Altman (2001) does provide an excellent overview of the complexity of this discussion.

The second major problem encountered is the choice of instrument used to measure disability. That is: what question(s) to ask in order to capture the proportion of disability in a population. In the past, many African countries have reported disability prevalence rates well under 5% (or below 5,000 per 100,000 population). This is far below the UN claim of 10% (see above) and rates observed in some western countries (the majority over 10%, some approaching 20%, Table 1). That is not to suggest that African rates should be as high as, or higher than those seen in western societies – but there is a real fear of under-reporting among African countries. What is lacking is a standardised approach to an evolving disability phenomenon so that international measurements can be compared.

The United Nations Statistical Division acknowledges that data sources and methodologies used in the above table are country specific and that

Table 1. Prevalence (%) of Disability in Selected Countries.

	Year	%
High-income countries		
Canada	1991	15.5
Germany	1992	8.4
Italy	1994	5.0
Netherlands	1986	11.6
Norway	1991	33.0
Sweden	1988	12.1
Spain	1986	15.0
UK	1991	12.2
USA	1994	15.0
Low-income countries		
Kenya	1989	0.7
Malawi	1983	2.9
Namibia	1991	3.1
Nigeria	1991	0.5
Senegal	1988	1.1
South Africa	1980	0.5
Zambia	1990	0.9
Zimbabwe	1997	1.9

Source: Canada, Statistics Canada – Selected characteristics of persons with disabilities residing in households; Germany, Statistisches Bundesamt Wiesbaden, Population and labour market survey; Italy, Instituto Nazionale di Statistica; Netherlands, Central Bureau of Statistics and Netherlands Institute for Research on Social Welfare, Physical Disability; Norway, Statistics Norway – Survey of Level of Living; Sweden, Statistics Sweden; Spain, Encuesta Sobre Discapacidades, Deficiencias y Minusvalias; UK, Office of Population Censuses and Surveys; USA, United States Department of Health and Human Services, National Center for Health Statistics; Kenya, Central Bureau of Statistics, Kenya Population Census; Namibia, Central Statistical Office, 1991 Population and Housing Census; Nigeria, National Population Commission, 1991 Population Census; Senegal, Direction de la provision et de la statistique; South Africa, UNDP-ILO Report; Zambia, Central Statistical Office, Census of Population, Housing and Agriculture; Zimbabwe, Data are derived from a separate report, and are not available on the UNSD website.

precludes any comparability of prevalence rates among countries. Each of the surveys reported here used a different set of questions in order to identify persons with disabilities. In certain instances, disability screening questions are based on impairments while in others (see in particular, Norway) an activity limitation approach is employed. Some results are based on surveys and others on censuses. For more information see http://unstats.un.org/unsd/disability/ (UN, 2003).

Beyond these acknowledged discrepancies, what are the underlying reasons for the differences seen in disability prevalence rates between low- and high-income countries?

In September 2001, the United Nations Statistical Division organised a Workshop on Disability Statistics for Africa that was attended by representatives from 11 English-speaking African nations. Discussions focussed on issues of measuring disability prevalence. There was agreement that the figures reported for African countries reflected the most severe cases of disability in the population – and were in fact not dissimilar to rates for severe cases of disability reported in western countries. It was felt, however, that they failed to capture the mild to moderate degrees of disability or activity limitation/participation restriction. The cause of this omission may be simply that individuals do not acknowledge a limitation if they are unaware of the possibility of improving the situation with relatively simple technical aids.

Another plausible explanation for the discrepancy between low- and high-income countries may be found in an assessment of disability prevalence along the time axis. It is claimed that disability prevalence rates observed in the United States (and other high-income, western countries) in the 1950s were of about the same order of magnitude as those now observed in low-income countries; and that the rates we see in, for example, African states represent a manifestation of the delayed development of these countries (World Bank Disability Advisor, personal communication).

Other theories focus more on the socio-cultural determinants of disability. One can ask whether Euro-American desires for equality (understood as sameness or similarity) (Whyte & Ingstad, 1995) are reflected to the same degree in low-income cultures?

According to Whyte and Ingstad (1995), disability in the Euro-American arena exists within a framework of state, legal, economic and biomedical institutions. "In developing countries where (this kind of) institutional infrastructure exists only to a very limited degree, disability as a concept and an identity is not an explicit cultural concept. The meaning of impairment must be understood in terms of cosmology and values and purposes of social life." (Whyte & Ingstad, 1995, p. 10).

In many aboriginal African cultures, for example, disabled individuals are both integrated and accepted. Being identified through kinship, residence and rank or through membership to an age cohort is more important to social identity than is impairment (Talle, 1995).

Our understanding of disability as a condition and its associated infrastructure, i.e. politics, human rights, law, policy, economy, education, professionalism, etc. are defined by our own socio-cultural perspective. We are likewise obliged to acknowledge and accept other socio-cultural perspectives and their influence on shaping disability cross-culturally.

In attempting to determine the amount of disability in a society, we are thus forced to examine that society's attitude towards disability and the *coping mechanisms* or capabilities of people with disabilities in society. We may ask, in other words, what do people with disabilities expect from society and what demands does society place on them? It is postulated that the extent of demands society places on the individual with a disability is directly proportional to the prevalence of disability in society (i.e. the more society demands, the more disability). But we must also take into account the ability of the person with a disability.

Disability can be measured as the gap between that which society demands and that which a person is able to manage. The more society demands of the individual with a disability the less that individual will be able to manage thereby resulting in more recorded cases of disability. Even in "healthy" Norway we can document an increase in the number of persons unemployed or on disability pension as the demands of business, industry and society on the individual increase over and beyond the individual's capabilities (both physical and psychological).

Conversely, in less techno-dependent, non-western societies, reading and writing difficulties may, for example, "not exist" mainly because society places fewer demands on individuals.

By altering society's notion of disability – from the concept of physical impairment to one based on activities and participation – it is hoped to shift also the focus of demands set by society while at the same time empowering the person with a disability. Research on living conditions among people with disabilities must ultimately be directed towards the integration, participation and enfranchisement of people with disabilities into society.

PURPOSE OF CURRENT STUDIES IN SOUTHERN AFRICA

The situation for people with disabilities in low-income countries is of concern for Governments, Non-Governmental Organisations (NGO), as well as for the International Community. Their rights have been the subject of much attention in the United Nations and other international organisations over a long period of time. The International Year of Disabled Persons (1981) and the United Nations Decade of Disabled Persons (1983–1992) culminated in the World Programme of Action Concerning Disabled Persons

(UN, 1982). The Programme emphasises the right of persons with disabilities to the same opportunities as other citizens and to an equal share in the improvements in living conditions resulting from economic and social development. In 1993, the General Assembly approved The Standard Rules on the Equalisation of Opportunities for Persons with Disabilities (Resolution 48/96) (UN, 1994), setting specific targets and requesting a strong moral and political commitment on behalf of States to take action for the equalisation of opportunities for persons with disabilities.

Knowledge about the living conditions among people with disabilities is important as a tool for advocacy and practical action, when agreeing on acceptable standards, setting priorities and planning for required improvements. Without the necessary information and knowledge, Governments, NGOs and International Organisations are more or less forced to work arbitrarily on a hit-or-miss basis. Under such circumstances resources cannot be distributed and utilised in a rational, efficient manner. Unfortunately, the lack of knowledge is clearly most pronounced in low-income countries with scarce resources and thus with the greatest need for cost-effective strategies that would improve the living conditions among people with disabilities.

With this backdrop, we launched in 2001 the first of to-date three national, representative surveys to quantify the living conditions among people with disabilities in southern Africa (Namibia: Eide, van Rooy, & Loeb, 2003a; Zimbabwe: Eide, Nhiwaitiwa, Muderedzi, & Loeb, 2003b; Malawi: Loeb & Eide, 2004). Specifically, the objectives for the surveys were:

1. to develop a strategy and methodology for the collection of comprehensive, reliable and culturally adapted statistical data on living conditions among people with disabilities.
2. to provide organizations for people with disabilities as well as local, regional and national authorities with up-to-date documentation on the state of living conditions among people with disabilities.
3. to include and involve people with disability in every step of the research process.
4. to initiate a discussion on the concepts and understanding of "disability," in particular in the perspective of developing countries.

DESIGN AND METHODS

The design that has been developed and tested in these studies aims at combining two research traditions: studies on living conditions and disability studies.[2] Pre-existing and validated questionnaires that had been previously used in Namibia (on general living conditions – NPC, 2000) and in South Africa (on disability – Schneider et al., 1999) were combined and adapted for use in the surveys. A third element, on activity limitations and participation restrictions, was included to incorporate the conceptual developments that have taken place in connection with the ICF.

The questionnaires used in these surveys were comprehensive,[3] and in each country a Reference Group of key stakeholders including national organisations of people with disabilities, representatives from government ministries and NGOs was established to discuss the questionnaire design and content and ensure that individual questions were suitably adapted to local cultures.

From the onset, the target population for sampling was all private households excluding institutionalised and homeless people. Trained enumerators in each country conducted household interviews with an identified head of household. Sample sizes in the three country surveys were: Namibia, 3,642 households, 23,314 individuals; Zimbabwe,[4] 3,901 households, 21,712 individuals; Malawi, 3,058 households, 15,364 individuals. Specific details of study design in each country as well as sampling methodologies and interview procedures are available in published reports online at http://www.sintef.no/content/page1_1561.aspx. Copies of the questionnaires used are available from the authors.

The approach used to screen for disability in the surveys undertaken in southern Africa relied on an understanding of disability as difficulties in doing day-to-day activities and/or restrictions in social participation. The screening questions used reflect an understanding of disability in accordance with the ICF (WHO, 2001b).

> Screening question 1. Does anyone in this household ever have any difficulty in doing day-to-day activities because of a physical, mental or emotional (or other health) condition which has lasted or is expected to last for six months or more? (Response categories: yes, no).
>
> Screening question 2. Does anyone in this household need assistance in participating in any of the following activities? (walking, seeing, speaking, hearing, breathing, mental coping, learning/comprehending) (Response categories: yes, no).

As a classification, the ICF can further be used to describe the process of functioning and disability by providing the means to map the different constructs and domains. The ICF provides a multi-perspective approach to the classification of functioning and disability as an interactive and evolutionary process.

In order to operationalise the ICF in a large survey, we developed a matrix that was intended to capture as many of the constructs as possible in a simple and non-time-consuming manner (see the appendix). The matrix attempts to capture activity limitations and participation restrictions through two questions:

1. How difficult is it for you to perform this activity without any kind of assistance at all? (that is, without the use of any assistive devices – either technical or personal).
2. Do you experience any problem(s) in performing this activity in your current environment? (*Current environment* refers to the surroundings in which one lives, works, plays, etc. for the majority of their time.)

These questions are asked with reference to 44 specific activities in nine categories. In addition to mapping an individual's degree of activity limitations and participation restrictions, determinants of a person's environment are sought through the categorising of facilitators and/or barriers that they may come up against with respect to those activity limitations/participation restrictions they experience.

UNDERSTANDING THE ACTIVITY LIMITATION AND PARTICIPATION RESTRICTION MATRIX

It is important to be able to differentiate between the two concepts or dimensions that we have attempted to capture by using this ICF-based matrix. While on the surface activity limitations and participation restrictions may appear similar, they do in fact measure two distinct aspects of the disability phenomenon. In considering *activity limitations* we ask: "How difficult is it for you to perform this activity *without any kind of assistance at all*?" The intention is to capture or measure an individual's *capacity* to carry out the 44 different activities of daily living listed in the matrix – it is a measure of the person's level of functioning. *Participation restrictions*, on the other hand, measure an individual's level of *performance* in their current or usual environment (i.e. where they normally are: at home, at school or at work). To capture this aspect we ask: "Do you experience any problem(s) in performing this activity in your *current environment*?"

A few simple examples may help to clarify this better.

1. A young boy lost the use of his legs in an automobile accident 25 years ago. He has been confined to a wheelchair since being discharged from the

hospital. Today he is an active member of society, working and supporting a family. Because he is dependent on the wheelchair, his scores on certain elements in the matrix will be high: he cannot move about easily without assistance. At the same time this person has become accustomed to life in a wheelchair, and in his current environment he is able to get around with little hindrance – he will score lower on the scale of participation restrictions.
2. Consider two individuals, 20 years old, both of whom are blind. One was born without the benefit of sight and the other became blind 6 months ago as a result of a work-related accident. Both have identical impairments and their activity limitations will, for the most part be the same – but the person who was born blind has had the benefit of 20 years to live with that condition – and in fact has never experienced living with sight. That person may be able to carry out all or most of their activities of daily living with little or no problem. The person who has been experiencing blindness for only 6 months may be quite helpless in their current environment.

We find that if disability is measured according to some predefined societal norm then we neglect to take into account the individual's own experiences (interacting with their social and physical environment) with respect to their particular disability. Measurements should rather be based on an individual's experience and capability in their environment.

DATA ANALYSIS

All questionnaires were controlled and signed by a trained supervisor upon completion of the interview. Completed questionnaires were transported to the local collaborating university centres for data cleaning and entry. Data were entered into SPSS data files and upon completion of data entry and data control, the data files were relayed to Norway and furthered analysed using SPSS 11.0. The significance of observed differences between variables presented here was tested using an analysis of variance (F statistic). A difference was considered to be statistically significant if $p<0.05$.

RESULTS

Measures of Activity Limitations and Participation Restrictions

The matrix described above is intended to map an individual's activity limitations and participation restrictions according to different parameters or domains: sensory experiences, basic learning and applying knowledge, communication, mobility, self care, domestic life, interpersonal behaviours, major life areas and community, social and civic life. For each item or activity under these nine parameters the degree to which an individual was capable of carrying out the activity without assistance (perceived activity limitation) was recorded on a scale from (0) no difficulty to (4) unable to carry out the activity. In the same manner, the person's performance in their current environment (perceived degree of participation restriction) was also recorded on a scale from (0) no problem to (4) unable to perform the activity. Based on the recorded observations for each of the 44 items a single activity limitation score and participation restriction score was developed as the sum of all 44 items (maximum possible score 176). The activity limitation score ranged from 0 to 155 (mean 29.2, median 22.0, standard deviation 24.8) and the participation restriction score ranged from 0 to 154 (mean 23.0, median 16.0, standard deviation 22.5).

These measures were assessed by type of impairment. (Results are presented for the Malawian survey; results from Namibia and Zimbabwe were similar.)

The results of the analysis of variance in Table 2 showed that both the activity limitation score and the participation restriction score behaved similarly with respect to the type of disability – but they measure two separate and distinct aspects of living with a disability. The activity limitation score is a measure of an individual's capacity to carry out everyday activities without any form of assistance, and the participation restriction score measures an individual's ability to perform the same activities in their current environment (home, work or school). Mean scores for mental/emotional were, on both scales, significantly higher than scores for all other types of disabilities (Activity limitations: $F = 17.0$, $df = 3/1402$, $p<0.001$; Participation restrictions: $F = 17.1$, $df = 3/1391$, $p<0.001$). Generally speaking this indicates that individuals with mental/emotional disabilities experience significantly more barriers to full participation in society.

These measures of extent of disability were then assessed with respect to certain indicators of living conditions. We looked first at school attendance (re-coded: NO = never attended, and YES = currently attending/left school). Mean scores based on activity limitations and participation restrictions showed that those who never had attended school scored higher (experienced greater activity limitations and restrictions to full participation in society) (Table 3).

We then addressed work situation for those 15 years of age or higher (re-coded: currently employed, previously employed, never been employed and housewife) (Table 4). The scores based on activity limitations and

Table 2. Mean Scores by Type of Impairment.

	Type of Impairment			
	Seeing, hearing, communication	Mental/ emotional	Physical/ mobility	Age/other
Mean score based on	$n = 653$	$n = 189$	$n = 667$	$n = 57$
Activity limitations	24.8	39.1	31.1	26.9
Participation restrictions	19.3	32.7	24.3	19.0

Table 3. Mean Scores by School Attendance.

School Attendance (Age> = 5)	Never Attended	Currently Attending or Finished School		
Mean score based on	$n = 427$	$n = 795$	t Statistic	p Value
Activity limitations	34.4	25.5	5.5	<0.001
Participation restrictions	29.0	19.2	6.4	<0.001

participation restrictions again showed similar patterns. Both showed that those who are currently employed scored lowest: this again can be seen as a validation of the two scores in that the ability to work represents a situation of less activity limitation and greater social participation. Housewives score lower than those not currently or never employed again reflecting to a degree their level of activity and social participation. The two groups defined as not currently or never employed score highest on both scales; perhaps a reflection of the barriers they face in general.

Finally, a relatively small sub-sample of those in our Malawian sample who were identified through screening as NOT having a disability (405 individuals) was asked to complete the activities and participation matrix. Their responses (as sum scores) are illustrated in two figures (Figs. 1 and 2) together with sum scores for the sample identified as disabled.

The figures below clearly indicate that there is an overlap; that is, even people identified as not having a disability live with certain limitations in

Table 4. Mean Scores by Work Situation.

Work Situation (Age> = 15)	Currently Employed	Previously Employed	Never been Employed	Housewife		
Mean score based on	$n = 320$	$n = 195$	$n = 534$	$n = 72$	*F* Statistic	*p* Value
Activity limitations	20.5	35.5	34.0	28.9	22.4	<0.001
Participation restrictions	14.9	27.8	27.9	17.8	24.8	<0.001

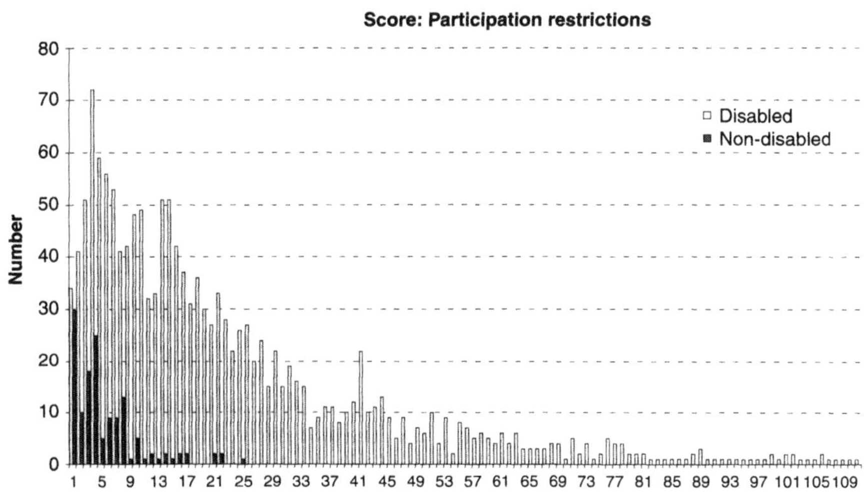

Fig. 1. Participation Restrictions among People with and without Disabilities.

their daily life activities and restrictions in their ability to participate in all levels of social interaction and some people with disabilities are able to function in society with little or no problem. While only 10 (0.6%) of those with disabilities scored 0 on the activity limitation scale compared to 63% of those without disabilities, it is important to stress that some of those people identified with disabilities are functioning well in society. Using the same reasoning we found that 37% of those individuals who were identified as not having a disability experienced at least a little problem in their capability to perform certain daily life activities.

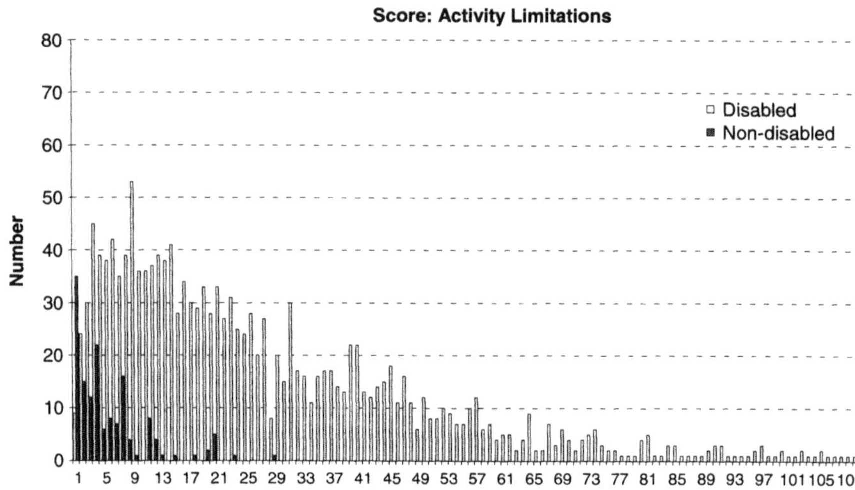

Fig. 2. Activity Limitations among People with and without Disabilities.

DISCUSSION

The results we present here, based on surveys undertaken in southern Africa, represent research in its infancy. Refinements to the tools used and improvements to the training of local enumerators and supervisors, in particular with respect to understanding the concepts of the ICF, will ultimately improve the precision, reliability and validity of the results achieved.

While results have been presented for Malawi only, both the Namibian and Zimbabwean surveys showed comparable findings. The questionnaires used in these surveys were comprehensive, and since input was solicited from each country with respect to adapting the questionnaires to local cultures, the data collected were not identical across the three countries and results at this stage cannot be seen as uniquely comparable.

It is interesting to note that participation restriction scores are lower than activity limitation scores. This is an indication that a person's capacity to perform activities in general – without assistance – (i.e. their activity limitations) is more restricted than their actual performance (participation restrictions). This is perhaps as might be expected, and is a reflection that many people with disabilities will have had at least some opportunity to adapt to their environments through, for example, the assistance of others or the use of different forms of assistive technology.

Also the range of scores on both activity limitations and participation restrictions reflects the diversity of disability in society – and clearly indicates that being disabled is not a singular, two-dimensional phenomenon but rather a complex process that deserves to be understood as part of the human condition and not as something that represents a deviation from the norm.

The determination of disability prevalence was not one of the original objectives of our research. We were, however, in a position to estimate prevalence based on the screening questions we used. As our approach to disability was based on activity limitations rather than impairments, we initially expected higher prevalence rates than those reported in earlier surveys (see Table 1) – but we found to our dismay that such was not the case. The prevalence of disability in Namibia, Zimbabwe and Malawi was estimated as 1.6%, 2.9% and 4.2% respectively (compared to 3.1%,[5] 1.9%[6] and 2.9%[7] recorded in previous surveys). Prevalence in Namibia was lower than previously recorded, in Zimbabwe marginally higher and approximately 45% higher in Malawi.

We accept these results as indicative, in part, of the evolving state of our experience both in terms of operationalising disability in research, and the complexity of the multi-cultural aspects of disability in low-income countries. All too often disability carries with it an ethno-cultural burden. No matter what language is used to approach the issue, stories of neglect, denial, discrimination and superstition are in its company. Even though we chose to approach disability through activity limitations and participation restrictions, our research was introduced at all levels as "Surveys of Living Conditions among People with *Disabilities*." What's in a name? Would that which we call *disability* by any other name smell as sweet? (with apologies to William Shakespeare, *Romeo and Juliet*, Act ii, Sc. 2).

CONCLUSIONS: TOWARDS A REVISED UNDERSTANDING OF DISABILITY

By altering society's notion of disability – from the concept of physical impairment to one based on activities and participation – it is hoped to shift also the focus of demands set by society while at the same time empowering people with disabilities. Research on living conditions among people with disabilities must ultimately be directed towards the integration, participation and enfranchisement of people with disabilities into society.

International standards are important for setting guidelines and establishing routines as much as for quantifying differences among nations, cultures and societies. But, at the same time, it is important not to become too fixated or restricted by these same international standards. A certain degree of flexibility must be allowed to be incorporated into these constructs. We are ultimately left with the following challenge: to acknowledge and integrate cultural anomalies and differences when making and interpreting international comparisons.

From the data analysis perspective, the research challenge, we believe, lies in a shift in the dependent variable from a dichotomous outcome measure (disabled, not disabled) to a continuous measure of activity limitation/participation restriction – mirroring the range of disability we see in society.

Finally, these measures of activity limitations and participation restrictions must be interpreted as relevant to the environment, society and culture from which they are derived. This will require an expanded view of disability data and effect substantially greater measurement challenges. We have in our research attempted to meet these challenges through the development of a matrix, based on the concepts inherent in the ICF.

NOTES

1. Low-income country will be applied throughout this article to cover terms like developing country, non-industrialised country, etc. Likewise, high-income country is applied to cover developed country, industrialised country, etc.
2. By "disability studies" we understand a broad specter of different studies that have generated knowledge about the situation of people with disabilities.
3. The questionnaire in its entirety is available from: mitch.loeb@sintef.no or arne.h.eide@sintef.no.
4. Due to the political and economic situation in Zimbabwe at the time of data collection, three regions (Matabeleland, Midlands and Manicaland) covering 5 of 10 provinces in the country and ca. 44% of the total population were surveyed.
5. Central Bureau of Statistics, 1991 Population and Housing Census, Namibia.
6. Central Statistical Office, 1997 Inter-Censal Demographic Survey Report, Zimbabwe.
7. National Statistical Office, 1987 Survey of Handicapped Persons, Malawi.

REFERENCES

Altman, B. M. (2001). Disability definitions, models, classification schemes and applications. In: G. L. Albrecht, K. D. Seelman & M. Bury (Eds), *Handbook of disability studies*. London: Sage Publications Inc.

Eide, A. H., Nhiwaitiwa, S., Muderedzi, J., & Loeb, M. E. (2003b). *Living conditions among people with activity limitations in Zimbabwe. A representative, regional study.* STF78 A034512. SINTEF Unimed NIS Health & Rehabilitation, Oslo.

Eide, A. H., van Rooy, G., & Loeb, M. (2003a). *Living conditions among people with disabilities in Namibia. A national, representative study*. STF78 A034503. SINTEF Unimed Health & Rehabilitation, Oslo.

Loeb, M., & Eide, A. H. (2004). *Living conditions among people with activity limitations in Malawi: A national representative study*. STF78 A044511. SINTEF Health Research, Oslo.

NPC – National Planning Commission. (2000). *Level of living conditions survey*. Planning Commission, Windhoek.

Schneider, M., Claassens, M., Kimmie, Z., Morgan, R., Naicker, S., Roberts, A., & McLaren, P. (1999). *We also count! The extent of moderate and severe reported disability and the nature of disability experience in South Africa*. Pretoria: Community Agency for Social Enquiry.

Talle, A. (1995). A child is a child: Disability and equality among the Kenya Maasai. In: B. Ingstad & S. R. Whyte (Eds), *Disability and culture*. London: University of California Press.

United Nations (UN). (1982). *World programme of action concerning disabled persons*. A/RES/37/52, New York: United Nations.

United Nations (UN). (1994). *The standard rules on the equalization of opportunities for persons with disabilities*. New York: United Nations.

United Nations (UN). (2003). http://unstats.un.org/unsd/disability/

Whyte, S. R., & Ingstad, B. (1995). Disability and culture: An overview. In: B. Ingstad & S. R. Whyte (Eds), *Disability and culture*. London: University of California Press.

World Health Organisation (WHO). (2001a). *WHO publishes new guidelines to measure health*. Press Release WHO/48. Geneva: World Health Organisation.

World Health Organisation (WHO). (2001b). *International classification of functioning, disability and health: ICF*. Geneva: World Health Organisation.

APPENDIX. ACTIVITY AND PARTICIPATION MATRIX

ACTIVITIES & PARTICIPATION Identification of person with disability: Name: .... Line No.:	Activity limitation (Capacity) 0 no difficulty 1 mild difficulty 2 moderate difficulty 3 severe difficulty 4 unable to carry out the activity 8 not applicable 9 not specified (level not known)	Participation restriction (Performance in current environment*) 0 no problem 1 mild problem 2 moderate problem 3 severe problem 4 complete problem (unable to perform) 8 not applicable 9 not specified (level not known)
a. watching/looking		
b. listening/hearing		
a. learning to read/write/count/calculate		
b. acquiring skills (manipulating tools, learning names)		
c. thinking		
d. reading/writing/counting/calculating		
e. solving problems		
a. understanding others (spoken, written or sign language)		
b. producing messages (spoken, written or sign language)		
c. communicating with others		
d. communicating using devices (phone/typewriter/computer/Braille)		
a. staying in one body position		
b. changing a body position (sitting/standing/bending/lying)		
c. transferring oneself (moving from one surface to another)		
d. lifting/carrying/moving/handling objects		
e. fine hand use (picking up/grasping/manipulating/releasing)		
f. hand & arm use pulling/pushing/reaching/throwing/catching		
g. walking		
h. moving around (crawling/climbing/running/jumping)		
i. moving around using equipment/assistive devices		
j. using transportation to move around as a passenger		
k. driving a vehicle (car/boat/bicycle/or riding an animal)		
a. washing oneself		
b. care of body parts, teeth, nails and hair		
c. toileting		
d. dressing and undressing		
e. eating and drinking		
a. shopping (getting goods and services)		
b. preparing meals		
c. doing housework (washing/cleaning)		
d. taking care of personal objects (mending/repairing)		
e. taking care of others		
a. making friends and maintaining friendships		
b. interacting with persons in authority		
c. interacting with strangers		
d. creating and maintaining family relationships		
e. creating and maintaining intimate relationships		
a. going to school and studying (education)		
b. getting and keeping a job (work & employment)		
c. handling income and payments (economic life)		
a. clubs/organisations (community life)		
b. recreation/leisure (sports/play/crafts/hobbies/arts/culture)		
c. religious/spiritual activities		
d. political life and citizenship		

**Your "current environment" is defined as where you spend most of your time: where you live, work, go to school or play.*

ENVIRONMENTAL FACTORS

1. **FACILITATORS: What makes it EASIER for you to participate? Think of things like products or devices, assistive technology, personal support, services, systems, policies, even attitudes – and tell me specifically what these might be.** *(Write down what respondent says in their own words.)*

   ____

   ____

2. **BARRIERS: What makes it HARDER for you to participate? Think of things like products or devices, assistive technology, personal support, services, systems, policies, even attitudes – and tell me specifically what these might be.** *(Write down what respondent says in their own words.)*

   ____

   ____

PEOPLE WITH DISABILITY IN BRAZIL: A LOOK AT 2000 CENSUS RESULTS

Alicia Bercovich

ABSTRACT

A new measure of disability used in the 2000 Census allows an expanded data set on the population with disabilities within all regions of Brazil. Using two different conceptualizations of disability including limitations in activities and impairments in body function and structure, the questions provide a richer source of information for policy issues. Initial use of the data has provided increased knowledge about the age, sex and racial makeup of the populations with disabilities and the geographic distribution of this population within Brazil.

INTRODUCTION

Questions related to people with disability were included in the Brazilian Decennial Censuses from 1872 to 1940. In the second half of the 20th century, they were excluded from the Census Forms. However, the enactment of Law No. 7.853 dated October 24, 1989 (Brazil, 1989) brought, among

International Views on Disability Measures: Moving Toward Comparative Measurement
Research in Social Science and Disability, Volume 4, 131–158

ISSN: 1479-3547/doi:10.1016/S1479-3547(05)04009-1

other legal guarantees, the obligation of including specific questions on people with disability in the national censuses. The information on this theme had become an indispensable condition for supporting the definition of policies adequate to the national context. Since 1991, the Brazilian Censuses include a set of questions on disability.

In the 2000 Census the questions that were formulated allowed the study of the people with disabilities, the starting point was to identify activity limitation and the degree of severity. Formulation of the questions was the product of a joint effort between the *Instituto Brasileiro de Geografia e Estatística* (IBGE) and the *Coordenadoria Nacional para Integração da Pessoa Portadora de Deficiência* (CORDE), of the Brazilian Government. The 2000 Census questions on disability permitted the study of the perception that the individuals have in relation to the changes caused by the disability on their realized capabilities, behavior and social participation.

To arrive at the formulation used, several pilot tests were performed with different sets of questions to select those that best identified the population being studied. The analyses of the results of these tests, together with the application of international experience, led to the questions applied in the 2000 Census. Some questions use the concept of limitation of activities to identify the disabilities. Two other questions refer to the impairments reflected in body functions and structures. The concept used, includes various levels of limitation of activities that enable the degrees of severity of limitation with vision, hearing and locomotion to be distinguished.

These conceptual bases are compatible with international recommendations, especially the International Classification of Functioning, Disability and Health (ICF) unveiled recently by the World Health Organization (WHO, 2001). The United Nations recommends the international classification to be used as a theoretical benchmark, and its concepts and terminology to provide international language that allows comparability of the statistics produced, whenever they attend to the information needs of each country (Mbogoni & Synneborn, 2003). Currently disability statistics vary noticeably between different countries, since they depend on the concepts used to develop measures in each country. The purpose is to harmonize concepts to arrive at a comparable data set between countries.

Several analyses were performed with the Brazil 2000 Census data to evaluate the consistency of the relationship between disability and vulnerability. In Table 1 the proportion of population with disability for a set of selected countries can be observed. The rates obtained are in decreasing order, showing the diversity of the concepts and measures used.

Table 1. Prevalence of Disability in Selected Countries by Source.

Country	Year	Proportion of Population with Disability (%)	Source
New Zealand	2001	19.5	Survey
United States of America	2000	19.3	Census
Australia	1998	19.0	Survey
United Kingdom	2001	17.6	Census
Brazil	2000	14.5	Census
Austria	1986	14.4	Survey
Italy	1999–2000	13.0	Survey
Sweden	1988	12.1	Survey
Netherlands	1986	11.6	Survey
Canada	2001	11.5	Census
Uruguay	2003–2004	11.0	Survey
Poland	1988	9.9	Census
Spain	1999	9.0	Survey
Germany	1992	8.4	Survey
China	1987	5.0	Survey
Chile	2002	2.2	Census
Mexico	2000	1.9	Census
Colombia	1993	1.8	Census

Source: United Nations Statistics Division; IBGE (Brazil); Bureau of the Census (USA); INEGI (Mexico); Statistics New Zealand, INE (Spain), AIHW (Australia) and INE (Uruguay).

The table shows the heterogeneity of measures and concepts used by different countries and the necessity of their harmonization.

AGE DISTRIBUTION AND STRUCTURE OF DISABILITY

Of the 24.6 million people with disability in Brazil (14.5% of the total population), 19.8 million were located in urban areas and 4.8 million in rural areas in 2000. The percentage of people that declared that they had at least one type of impairment or limitation is 14.3% in the urban zones and 15.2% in the rural zones (IBGE, 2003). The southeast portion of the country is the region with the lowest proportion of people that declared themselves disabled (13.1%). However the Northeast has the highest percentage of disability, 16.8% (Table 2).

Table 2. Proportion of the Population with at least One Type of Disability, by Urban and Rural Area – Brazil and Regions 2000.

Regions	Proportion of the Population with at least One Type of Disability (%)		
	Total	Urban	Rural
Brazil	14.5	14.3	15.2
North	14.7	15.7	12.5
Northeast	16.8	17.0	16.3
Southeast	13.1	13.0	13.8
South	14.3	13.8	16.5
Central West	13.9	14.0	13.1

Source: IBGE, 2000 Census.

Also considering the degree of severity of the impairment, it can be observed that there are 148,000 blind people in Brazil and 2.4 million people that declare that they have great difficulty in seeing. Of the total number of blind people, around 77,900 are women and 70,100 are men. Analogously 166,400 people declare themselves to be deaf, of which 80,000 are women and 86,400 are men. In Brazil almost 900,000 people declare that they have great permanent difficulty in hearing.

The regional distribution of the disabled population by type of impairment and degree of severity is shown in Table 3.

The Northeastern region, although its total population is lower than that of the Southeast, has approximately 57,400 people that declare themselves to be blind, against 54,600 in the Southeast.

Of the 166,400 people that declared themselves incapable of hearing in Brazil, approximately 60,000 live in the Southeastern region, while a 56,400 are located in the Northeastern region.

Analyzing the proportion of people with at least one type of impairment or disability according to age groups, it can be observed that in the case of children up to 14 years of age, 4.3% of them have at least one type of disability. This proportion increases to 15.6% of people of working age (aged 15–64). More than half of the people aged 65 or over declare that they have some type of impairment or disability. This proportion increases with age and is a consequence of the increase in the limitations on activities as a result of aging (Graph 1).

Analyzing this proportion at regional level, it can be seen that the North and Northeastern regions have the largest numbers of disabled people in all age groups. It is natural that as people become older, the proportion of them

Table 3. Population by Type of Disability and Sex – Brazil and Regions 2000.

Gender and Regions	Population													
	Total (1)(2)	Type of Disability												
		At least one type of disability	Permanent mental disability	Physical impairment	Seeing			Hearing			Mobility (3)			No disability
					Unable	Great permanent difficulty	Some permanent difficulty	Unable	Great permanent difficulty	Some permanent difficulty	Unable	Great permanent difficulty	Some permanent difficulty	
Brazil	169,872,856	24,600,256	2,844,937	1,416,060	148,023	2,435,873	14,060,946	166,365	883,079	4,685,655	574,186	1,772,690	5,592,908	143,726,947
North	12,911,170	1,901,892	189,902	107,526	11,061	205,173	1,199,136	13,259	56,083	320,088	36,377	98,906	371,237	10,870,702
Northeast	47,782,487	8,025,537	859,454	410,582	57,416	853,114	4,836,931	56,351	293,668	1,511,668	174,738	559,671	1,789,202	39,342,892
Southeast	72,430,193	9,459,596	1,201,606	586,526	54,600	863,101	5,113,771	59,991	335,929	1,823,400	243,417	733,630	2,259,819	62,262,577
South	25,110,348	3,595,028	409,783	215,313	17,562	355,348	1,953,350	24,460	139,720	734,303	85,173	280,414	845,394	21,343,756
Central West	11,638,658	1,618,204	184,192	96,113	7,384	159,139	957,757	12,304	57,680	296,196	34,481	100,069	327,255	9,907,021
Male	83,602,317	11,420,544	1,545,462	861,196	70,160	1,044,746	6,144,168	86,431	466,043	2,465,745	275,301	739,219	2,280,551	71,391,433
North	6,536,901	926,881	107,393	69,420	5,462	93,790	554,985	6,982	31,388	176,858	18,223	45,859	167,015	5,537,402
Northeast	23,430,808	3,645,185	472,056	245,258	26,854	365,977	2,065,519	29,655	154,273	752,907	80,497	234,560	727,891	19,575,913
Southeast	35,430,967	4,357,446	646,292	351,939	25,589	360,738	2,207,127	31,020	173,137	967,099	117,397	296,905	890,557	30,710,837
South	12,401,987	1,718,646	221,257	134,961	8,579	153,809	882,117	12,455	76,176	409,089	41,705	117,710	352,953	10,597,575
Central West	5,801,654	772,387	98,464	59,618	3,675	70,432	434,420	6,318	31,069	159,791	17,479	44,185	142,134	4,969,766
Female	86,270,539	13,179,712	1,299,474	554,864	77,863	1,391,127	7,916,778	79,934	417,037	2,219,910	298,885	1,033,471	3,312,357	72,335,514
North	6,374,269	975,012	82,508	38,105	5,599	111,383	644,151	6,277	24,696	143,230	18,155	53,047	204,222	5,333,301
Northeast	24,351,679	4,380,352	387,399	165,323	30,562	487,137	2,771,413	26,696	139,395	758,761	94,241	325,111	1,061,311	19,766,979
Southeast	36,999,226	5,102,150	555,314	234,588	29,011	502,362	2,906,645	28,971	162,792	856,300	126,020	436,725	1,369,262	31,551,739
South	12,708,361	1,876,382	188,525	80,353	8,983	201,538	1,071,233	12,004	63,543	325,213	43,467	162,705	492,441	10,746,240
Central West	5,837,004	84,5817	85,728	36,495	3,709	88,707	523,336	5,986	26,611	136,405	17,002	55,884	185,121	4,937,254

Source: IBGE, 2000 Census.

(1) People with more than one type of disability were counted only once. (2) Including people without answer to the questions on disability. (3) This means difficulty walking and climbing stairs.

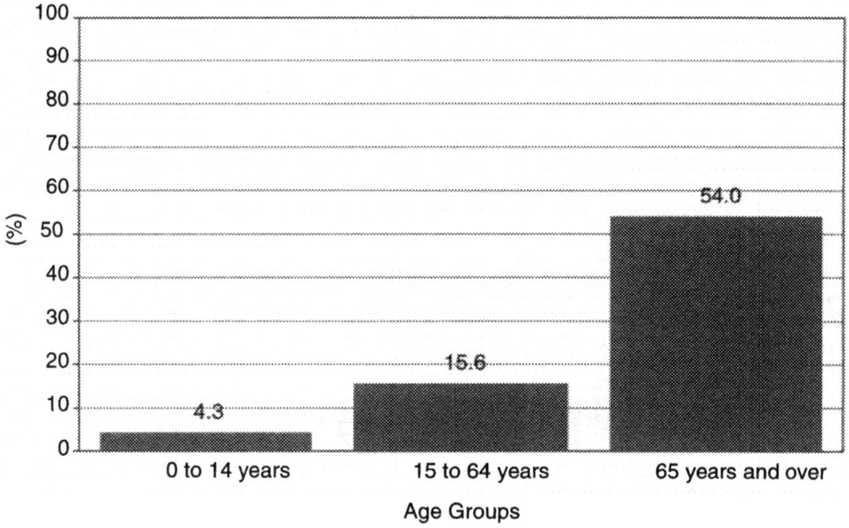

Graph 1. Proportion of the Population with at least One Type of Disability, by Age Groups, Brazil 2000. *Source:* IBGE, 2000 Census.

Table 4. Proportion of the Population with at least One Type of Disability, by Special Age Groups – Brazil and Regions 2000.

Regions	Proportion of the Population with at least One Type of Disability (%)			
	Total	0–14 years old	15–64 years old	65 years old and over
Brazil	14.5	4.3	15.6	54.0
North	14.7	4.6	18.1	63.2
Northeast	16.8	5.2	18.7	62.3
Southeast	13.1	3.7	13.5	48.0
South	14.3	3.7	15.1	53.5
Central West	13.9	4.4	15.5	56.2

Source: IBGE, 2000 Census.

with at least some difficulty with vision, hearing or locomotion increases (Table 4).

The male mortality rate is higher than the female rate for age groups, and therefore an important part of the disabled population aged 65 and over is made up of women.

When analyzing the proportion of people with at least one disability according to their individual ages, two points of inflection or ages at which the proportion increases can be observed: the first as from the age of 10 and the second from 40.

The first point of inflection is related with the entry of children into the school system, and the increase in perception of certain disabilities as a result of difficulties in performing school activities. On the other hand as from age 40, the problem is related with aging and the increasing difficulty to see, hear or walk (Graph 2).

When observing the composition of the age pyramid of the total number of people with at least one type of disability, it was found that the largest absolute number of disabled people was in the population between the ages of 40 and 49, especially females. In Brazil there are almost 4.5 million people between the ages of 40 and 49 with at least one type of impairment or disability, of which 2.4 million are women and almost 2.1 million are men. In this case the group of people with at least some difficulty in seeing predominates.

In the case of difficulties in hearing or walking, the most numerous groups are the ages between 60 and 69 (Graph 3).

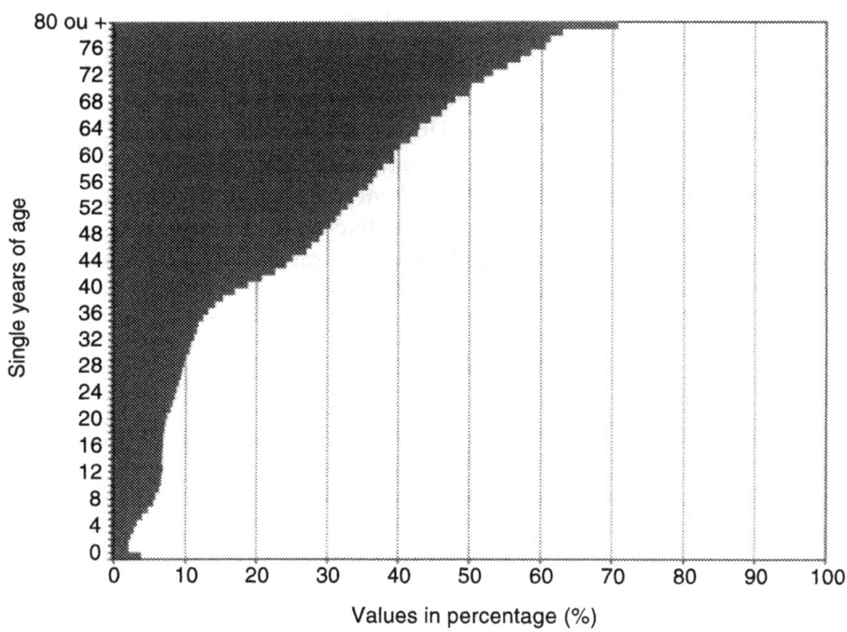

Graph 2. Proportion of the Population with at least One Type of Disability, by Single Years of Age, Brazil –2000. *Source:* IBGE, 2000 Census.

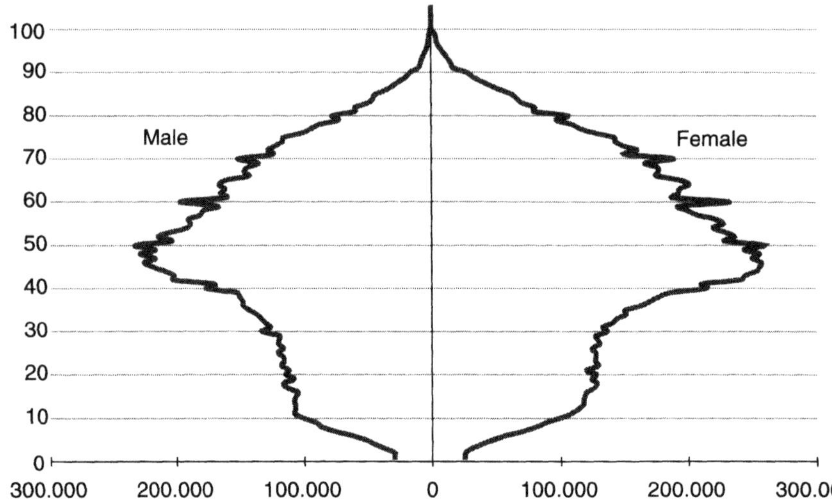

Graph 3. Age and Sex Structure of the Population with at least One Type of Disability, Brazil 2000. *Source:* IBGE, 2000 Census.

When analyzing the sex ratio of people with at least one type of disability, it can be seen that the sex ratio of the disabled population reduces as from the age of 50, in other words the proportion of women with at least one type of impairment or disability increases. The sex ratio in the Brazilian population is 96.9 men for each 100 women. Among disabled people there are only 86.7 men for each 100 women. This difference increases in the urban zones (94.1% and 82.7% for men per 100 women respectively). In the rural zones, the men always predominate, 110.1 men for each 100 women in total, and only 104.6 men per 100 women are found in the disabled group (Table 5).

RACE AND ETHNICITY

Considering color or race in estimating the prevalence of disability, it can be observed that the largest prevalence of disability can be found in the population that (Table 6) declares itself to be black, and lower in the population that declares itself to be white.

At the regional level the lower prevalence of disability corresponds to the white population in the Southeast (12.6%) and the higher is for black people (19.6%) in the Northeast. Once again the relationship between the socio-economic characteristics of the population and the prevalence of disability can be observed.

Table 5. Sex Ratio in Population with and without Disability by Urban and Rural Area Brazil and Regions 2000.

Regions	Sex Ratio					
	Total		Urban		Rural	
	Total	With at least one type of disability	Total	With at least one type of disability	Total	With at least one type of disability
Brazil	96.9	86.7	94.1	82.7	110.1	104.6
North	102.6	95.1	97.1	87.0	116.4	122.9
Northeast	96.2	83.2	91.7	77.5	107.1	98.2
Southeast	95.8	85.4	94.3	83.3	111.1	106.2
South	97.6	91.6	94.9	87.6	109.8	107.4
Central West	99.4	91.3	96.5	87.0	120.6	128.0

Source: IBGE, 2000 Census.

Table 6. Proportion of the Population with at least One Disability, by Colour/Race Brazil and Regions 2000.

Regions	Proportion of the Population with at least One Type of Disability (%)					
	Total	White	Black	Yellow	Mixed	Indigenous
Brazil	14.5	13.8	17.5	13.9	15.0	17.1
North	14.7	14.7	18.1	15.6	14.6	10.6
Northeast	16.8	16.8	19.6	18.3	16.4	21.5
Southeast	13.1	12.6	15.8	13.1	13.5	21.7
South	14.3	14.1	16.6	14.3	15.4	19.5
Central West	13.9	13.5	18.3	15.2	13.9	13.7

Source: IBGE, 2000 Census.

LITERACY

It can be observed that the literacy rate for people of 15 years of age or more in Brazil is 87.1%. Among disabled people this proportion falls to 72.0%. If we consider only severe disabilities[1] the proportion of literate people of more than 15 years of age falls to 61.6%. In the case of the Northeast, almost half the people with severe impairments or disabilities (46.7%) were literate (Table 7) (Graph 4).

Table 7. Literacy Rate Among Adults Aged 15 Years and over in Population with and without Disability – Brazil and Regions 2000.

Regions	Literacy Rate among Adults Aged 15 Years Old and Over (%)		
	Total (1) (2)	At least one type of disability	At least one type of severe disability (3)
Brazil	87.1	72.0	61.6
North	84.3	71.6	59.5
Northeast	75.1	57.9	46.7
Southeast	92.3	79.8	69.8
South	92.8	81.1	70.9
Central West	89.8	75.0	63.3

Source: IBGE, 2000 Census.

(1) People with more than one type of disability were counted only once. (2) Including people without answer to the questions on disability. (3) Excluding people with some permanent difficulty to see, hear, walk or climb stairs.

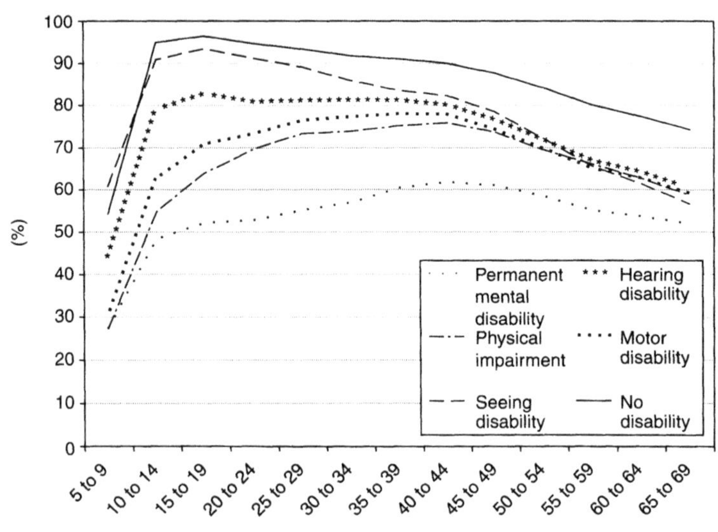

Graph 4. Proportion of Literate People Aged 5 Years and over by Type of Disability and Age Groups, Brazil 2000. *Source:* IBGE, 2000 Census.

When considering the literacy rates by age group and type of disability, it can be observed that mental disability and partial or total paralysis are related with lower literacy rates.

The people with at least some difficulty in seeing are those that have the highest literacy rates and are most similar to those that have none of the impairments or disabilities investigated.

SCHOOL ATTENDANCE

The fact of having at least one disability reduces school attendance even in the age range when this is mandatory by law.

The attendance of children aged between 7 and 14 with disabilities is 88.6%; therefore six percentage points below the school attendance rate of children in this age group, which is 94.5%. The same tendency is observed for most of the regions and the difference between the rates is of the same magnitude as the rate for Brazil. It is important to highlight that a significant portion of disabled children attend regular lessons; only some of them are considered to have special needs and receive supplementary attention or are enrolled at special schools. There is evidence that disabled children learn better when they attend regular schools in the community. Several studies and various international organizations such as UNESCO and the OECD have found that inclusive education is the best route to educate students with special needs (Porter, 2001).

It is obvious that it is not sufficient to enroll part of the disabled children in regular education, it is also necessary for the educators to be prepared to effectively (Table 8) integrate the students into the system.

Observing the attendance rates of children aged between 7 and 14 and the type of disability in the case of Brazil, it can be noted that the problems responsible for the lowest rates of school attendance of children are physical impairments (61%) and permanent mental impairments (66.5%). Children with visual impairments are less affected as regards school attendance, with 93.3% at school for an overall rate of 95% in the case of children that declare they have none of the impairments investigated (Table 9).

The rate of school attendance for children with each type of disability and age group confirms that children with permanent physical disabilities have a lower attendance rate and those with visual impairments are those whose rate of attendance is closest to people who declare that they do not have any of the disabilities investigated. It can be observed that the rate of school attendance by age group, even at the maximum point of the curve, for

Table 8. School Attendance Rate among Children Aged 7 to 14 Years with and without Disability – Brazil and Regions 2000.

Regions	School Attendance Rate among Children Aged 7 to 14 Years (%)		
	Total (1) (2)	At least one type of disability	At least one type of severity disability (3)
Brazil	94.5	88.6	74.9
North	88.8	86.8	71.5
Northeast	92.9	87.5	69.9
Southeast	96.3	89.7	78.2
South	96.5	89.7	78.7
Central West	95.5	90.9	79.5

Source: IBGE, 2000 Census.
(1) People with more than one type of disability were counted only once. (2) Including people without answer to the questions on disability. (3) Excluding people with some permanent difficulty to see, hear, walk or climb stairs.

Table 9. School Attendance Rate among Children Aged 7 to 14 Years by Sex and Type of Disability – Brazil 2000.

Type of Disability	School Attendance Rate among Children Aged 7 to 14 Years		
	Total	Male	Female
Total (1)(2)	94.5	94.2	94.9
At least one type of disability	88.6	87.1	90.1
Permanent mental disability	66.5	65.8	67.3
Physical impairment	61.0	61.0	61.0
Unable, with some or great permanent difficulty seeing	93.3	92.5	94.0
Unable, with some or great permanent difficulty hearing	86.9	86.5	87.4
Unable, with some or great permanent difficulty hearing, walking or climbing stairs	70.3	68.9	71.9
No disability	94.9	94.7	95.2

Source: IBGE, 2000 Census.
(1) People with more than one type of disability were counted only once. (2) Including people without answer to the questions on disability.

children aged between 10 and 14 years is above 90%, and in the case of children with permanent physical or mental disabilities the attendance rate is just over 60%.

LEVEL OF EDUCATION

Table 10 shows the proportion of people aged 15 years and over, with at least one type of impairment or disability by years of schooling according to the regions of Brazil (Graph 5).

The first finding is that the differences in the prevalence of disability by level of education exceed any differences between the regions.

As was found for other demographic characteristics, the principal inflection points are the transition from no education and up to 3 years education to the subsequent level, and completion of the first grade, in other words 8 complete years of education. However, completion of the second grade does not seem to be a crucial factor in changing the prevalence of disability. It is important to stress that the difference between the percentage of those with disabilities in the group of people without education or with up to 3 years education, and the percentage corresponding to people with between 4 and 7 years of education

Table 10. Proportion of Population aged 15 Years and over, with at least One Type of Disability by Years of Schooling – Brazil and Regions 2000.

Regions	Proportion of Population Aged 15 Years and over, with at least One Type of Disability (%)				
	Total (1)	Years of Schooling Groups			
		Without education to 3 years	4–7 years	8–10 years	11 years and over
Brazil	18.8	32.9	16.7	10.7	10.1
North	20.7	30.7	16.6	13.6	14.1
Northeast	22.5	32.2	17.1	12.9	12.5
Southeast	16.5	32.7	16.2	9.8	9.1
South	18.4	37.5	18.2	9.8	9.0
Central West	18.0	33.5	15.5	10.6	10.2

Source: IBGE, 2000 Census.

(1) Including people with years of schooling not determinate.

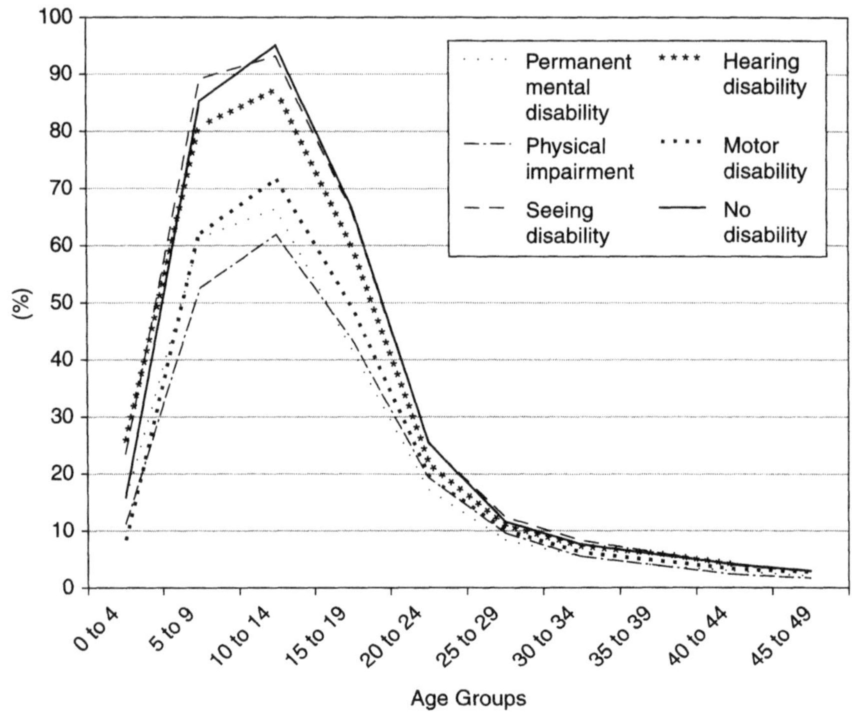

Graph 5. Proportion of People that Attend Nursery or School by Type of Disability and Age Groups Brazil 2000. *Source:* IBGE, 2000 Census.

exceeds 14 percentage points in all regions, while the difference between regions rarely exceeds five percentage points, and is much lower when the same proportions are observed for the same level of education. This shows the close correlation between the level of education and prevalence of disability.

SOCIOECONOMIC CHARACTERISTICS

The same trends and relationships between the level of education and disabilities are observed between the activity rates and occupation of people with disability.

In graphs 6 and 7 the rate of participation in economic activities of those without any and with at least one of the disabilities investigated can be observed (Graphs 6 and 7).

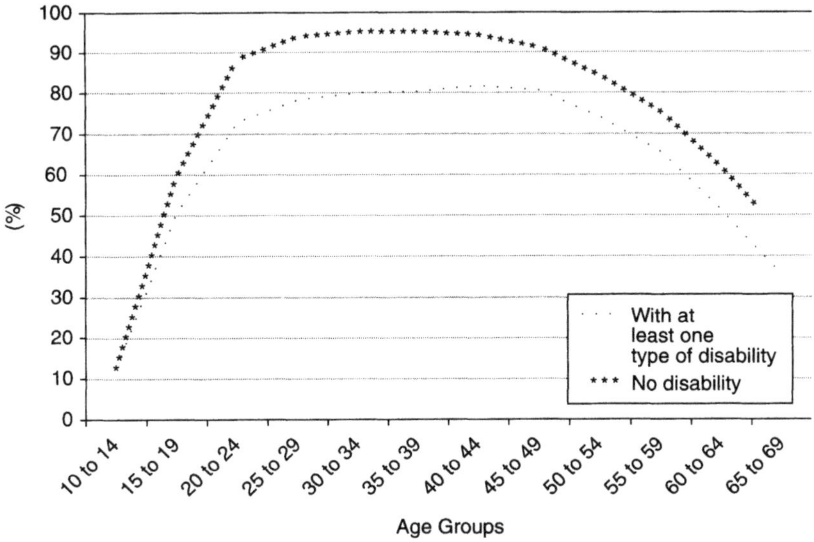

Graph 6. Labor Force Participation Rate of People with and without Disability, by Age Groups – Males Brazil 2000. *Source:* IBGE, 2000 Census.

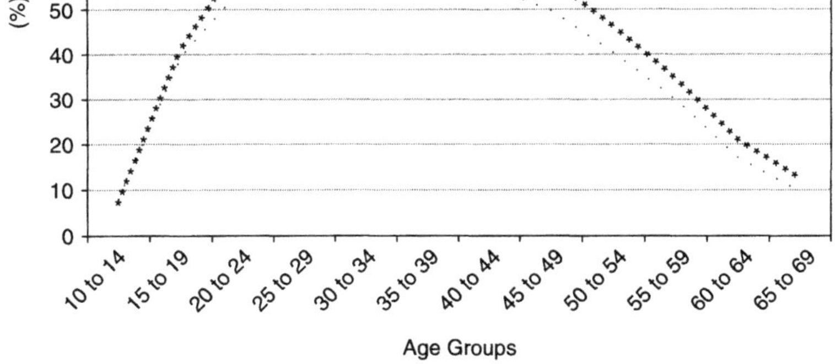

Graph 7. Labor Force Participation Rate of People with and without Disability, by Age Groups – Females Brazil 2000. *Source:* IBGE, 2000 Census.

As always, female activity rates are lower than the male rates, but the differences between the sexes are greater than between being disabled or not. The difference between the sexes for the age groups with the highest rates of activities is of the order of 30 percentage points for people that declare that they have no disabilities and 20 percentage points for those with at least one disability. Montes and Massiah (2001) had shown similar results for Brazil, 1981. However, the 1981 survey used a different conceptual frame for disability.

On the other hand, the differences between the rates of male activity in the case of those with disabilities or not are around 15 percentage points and seven percentage points for females. The difference between those with or without disabilities affects males more than females.

When considering the types of disability, in graphs 8 and 9 it can be observed that the types of disability that most affect the activity rates are the same, and in the (Graphs 8 and 9) same order as for school attendance or level of education, with the exception of the physical and mental disabilities, which appear in the reverse order. Permanent mental impairment is the disability that most affects the activity rates, followed by physical and motor disabilities.

On the other hand vision or hearing problems are those that at least affect participation in the workforce. The rate of male participation, which is normally above 90% in the younger age group, does not exceed 40% for people with a mental disability in the same age groups.

Analogous results can be observed for the employment rates for each type of disability. In graphs 10 and 11 the employment rate for people with and without disabilities can be observed. Table 11 shows the employment rates by sex and type of disability. It is important to highlight that in the age groups with the highest proportion (Graphs 10 and 11) of working people, the employment rate of males with mental or physical disabilities is lower than that of women without any of the disabilities investigated (Table 12).

Analyzing the division of the occupied population among the various economic activities, it can be observed that similar to the results verified in other countries, many people that declare themselves to be disabled work in agriculture and related activities.

In particular 25% of the total number of people with at least one disability work in this kind of activity, while only 17% of the total number of occupied persons without any of the disabilities investigated works in these sectors.

On the other hand, also as expected, a relatively larger proportion of people without disabilities work in the transformation industry and commerce.

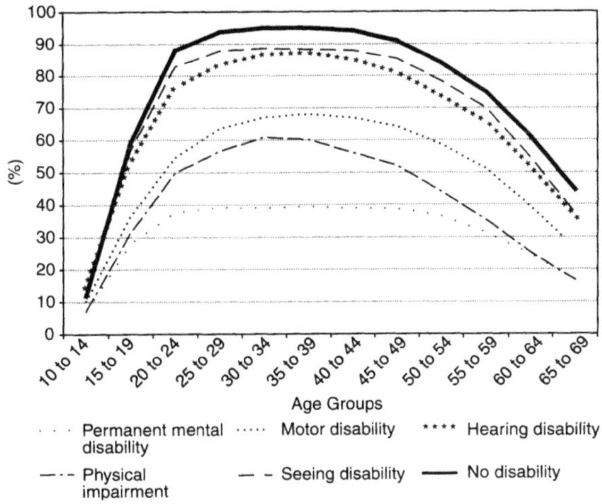

Graph 8. Labor Force Participation Rate of People with Disability, by Type of Disability and Age Groups – Males Brazil 2000. *Source:* IBGE, 2000 Census.

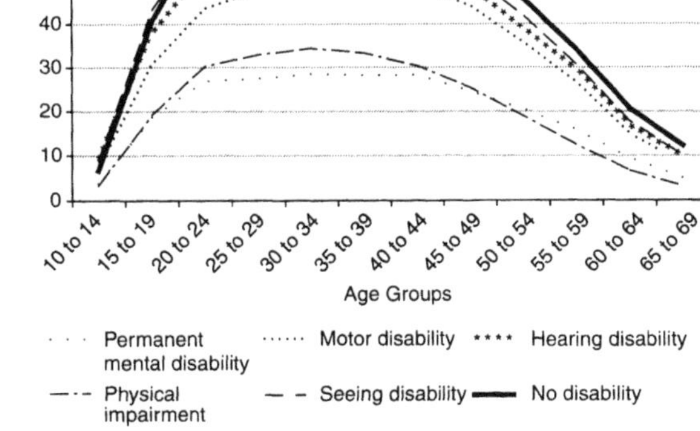

Graph 9. Labor Force Participation Rate of People with Disability, by Type of Disability and Age Groups – Females Brazil 2000. *Source:* IBGE, 2000 Census.

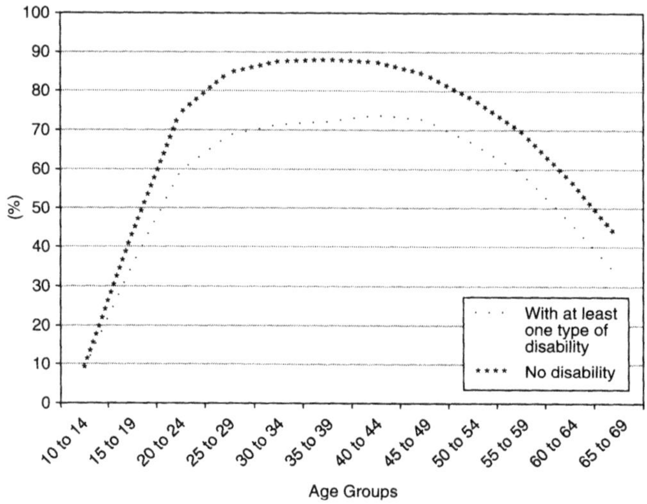

Graph. 10. Employment Rate of People with or without Disability, by Age Groups – Males Brazil 2000. *Source:* IBGE, 2000 Census.

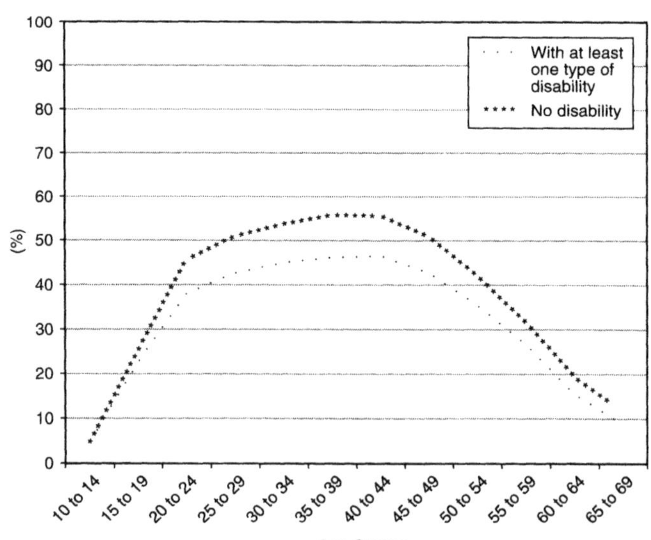

Graph 11. Employment Rate of People with or without Disability, by Age Groups – Females Brazil 2000. *Source:* IBGE, 2000 Census.

Table 11. Proportion of Employed People Aged 10 Years and over, in the Reference Week, by Type of Disability, Sex and Age Groups – Brazil 2000.

Age Groups (Years)	Proportion of Employed People Aged 10 Years Old and over in the Reference Week (%)													
	Male	Female	Type of Disability and Sex											
			No disability		Permanent mental disability		Physical impairment		Unable, with some or great permanent difficulty hearing, walking or climbing stairs		Unable, with some or great permanent difficulty seeing		Unable, with some or great permanent difficulty hearing	
			Male	Female	Male	Female	Male	Female	Male	Female	Male	Female	Male	Female
Total	61.1	35.4	63.0	37.2	24.2	13.7	31.9	11.9	34.8	18.0	55.9	29.2	45.9	20.7
10–14	8.8	4.3	8.8	4.3	5.1	2.3	5.4	1.9	7.1	4.1	9.7	5.3	10.1	5.0
15–19	41.9	24.6	42.4	24.8	19.3	11.1	22.1	11.0	24.5	17.3	39.0	24.3	37.1	22.0
15	24.0	12.7	24.2	12.6	12.6	5.8	12.7	6.7	15.7	10.1	23.6	14.6	25.0	12.2
16 ou 17	37.8	21.6	38.2	21.7	18.0	9.3	19.0	11.0	22.9	16.4	35.3	21.6	34.5	21.0
18 ou 19	54.6	33.4	55.4	33.7	23.8	15.3	29.3	13.1	30.0	21.6	49.8	31.6	46.1	27.7
20–24	72.9	44.7	74.0	45.3	28.8	18.8	40.2	21.2	43.2	28.6	68.0	41.6	62.2	35.1
25–29	82.9	49.9	84.4	50.7	31.6	20.9	48.5	23.7	53.4	34.8	77.5	46.2	72.8	41.4
30–34	85.5	52.6	87.2	53.5	32.2	22.2	53.1	26.9	57.9	38.3	79.7	48.2	77.0	44.4
35–39	85.7	54.2	87.7	55.5	33.1	22.1	52.8	26.9	59.0	40.4	79.7	48.9	78.1	46.5
40–44	84.5	53.3	87.1	55.2	33.5	22.7	49.9	25.5	58.2	39.6	79.5	48.2	75.8	45.9
45–49	81.0	48.4	84.1	50.6	33.2	20.3	45.5	21.3	55.6	36.7	77.1	44.0	71.0	40.6
50–54	74.2	39.7	77.5	41.7	31.6	17.1	38.8	16.0	51.1	30.4	70.7	36.7	64.7	33.6
55–59	65.7	29.6	69.3	31.3	27.6	13.7	31.3	10.9	44.9	23.2	63.3	27.4	58.0	25.7
60–64	52.7	17.5	56.9	19.0	21.5	8.1	22.6	5.6	34.9	13.0	49.8	15.9	45.7	14.3
65–69	37.6	10.1	41.8	11.3	15.1	4.3	15.1	2.7	23.6	7.2	34.2	9.0	32.3	8.4
70 and over	19.1	4.1	24.3	5.6	6.1	1.4	5.3	0.7	9.8	2.3	15.7	3.2	14.7	2.7

Source: IBGE, 2000 Census.

Table 12. Percentage Distribution of Employed People Aged 10 Years and over, in the Reference Week, by Type of Disability and Activity Section of the Primary Job – Brazil 2000.

Activity Sections of Primary Job	Percentage Distribution of Employed People Aged 10 Years and over in the Reference Week (%)								
	Total (1) (2)	Type of Disability							
		At least one type of disability	Permanent mental disability	Physical impairment		Unable, with some or great permanent difficulty seeing	Unable, with some or great permanent difficulty hearing	Unable, with some or great permanent difficulty hearing, working or climbing stairs	No disability
				Permanent tetraplegia, paraplegia or hemiplegia	Total or partial absence of limb (3)				
Total	100.0	100.0	100.0	100.0	100.0	100.0	100.0	100.0	100.0
Agriculture, hunting, forestry	17.9	25.0	26.8	19.6	24.7	26.2	26.7	27.0	16.8
Fishing	0.5	0.7	0.8	0.9	0.9	0.8	0.7	0.8	0.5
Mining and quarrying	0.4	0.4	0.4	0.3	0.6	0.3	0.5	0.3	0.4
Manufacturing	13.3	11.6	11.3	10.9	17.4	10.8	13.9	10.2	13.6
Electricity, gas and water supply	0.5	0.5	0.5	0.7	0.5	0.4	0.5	0.4	0.5
Construction	7.0	7.0	6.9	6.2	9.6	6.8	7.7	6.0	6.9
Wholesale and retail trade, repair of motor vehicles, motorcycles and personal and household goods	16.6	14.1	15.0	17.6	15.2	13.8	13.6	13.9	17.0

Hotels and restaurants	4.7	5.0	4.7	5.8	4.0	5.0	4.6	6.0	4.6
Transport, storage and communications	5.1	4.3	4.2	5.6	5.3	4.0	4.7	3.8	5.2
Financial Intermediation	1.3	0.7	0.9	0.7	0.6	0.7	0.6	0.5	1.3
Real Estate, renting and business activities	5.7	4.7	4.9	6.1	4.5	4.5	4.5	4.3	5.9
Public administration and defense, compulsory social security	5.4	5.1	4.4	5.9	4.1	5.2	4.8	4.9	5.4
Education	5.8	5.3	4.5	5.0	2.9	5.5	4.1	4.9	5.9
Health and social work	3.3	2.7	2.7	2.8	1.7	2.7	2.2	2.7	3.4
Other community, social and personal service activities	3.6	3.6	3.5	4.7	2.8	3.5	3.4	4.0	3.7
Activities of private households as employers and undifferentiated production activities of private households	7.6	8.0	7.0	5.5	3.8	8.4	6.2	9.1	7.6
Extra-territorial organizations and bodies	0.0	0.0	0.0	0.0	0.0	0.0	0.0	0.0	0.0
Activities not classified by field	1.3	1.3	1.5	1.6	1.4	1.3	1.3	1.3	1.3

Source: IBGE, 2000 Census.

(1) People with more than one type of disability were counted only once. (2) Including people without answer to the questions on disability. (3) Loss of a member: leg, arm, hand, foot or thumb.

An analogous situation can be observed with respect to occupational groups: disabled people constitute a larger proportion of workers in agriculture and cattle raising, forestry and related services.

The largest differences between the proportions of people occupied without disabilities and those with at least one disability are associated with workers in administrative services, medium level technicians and professionals in the sciences and arts fields. These results are compatible with those presented by Hernández-Licona (2001) for other countries. The distributions can be observed in Table 13.

The distribution of people occupied according to income in minimum salary ranges can be observed in Table 14.

The proportion of males that earns up to one minimum salary is 20.2%, while in the case of women the percentage is 28.5%. When people that declare they have at least one disability are considered, these proportions become 25.7% and 35.7% respectively. In the case of mental disability, 30.5% of the males and 33.1% of the females that work receive up to one minimum salary.

Throughout the study it is shown that disability and poverty are strictly related. The disability increases the probability of living under precarious conditions, which in turn increases the risk of acquiring a disability.

People with disability have lower levels of education, income and participation in the labor market. In addition, insertion in the workforce is mainly on occupations and activities that require a low degree of specialization. However this insertion varies according to the type of disability and the degree of severity.

DISABILITY-FREE LIFE EXPECTANCY

The significant increases in life expectancy that occurred during the 20th century have made chronic sicknesses and functional limitations more frequent, making the indicator, which is based exclusively on mortality, not entirely satisfactory to portray the health status of a population, as it did in the past.

As a result, the need arose for a measure that could expand the concept of life expectancy (LE) by including the individual ability to participate in society. The Disability-Free Life Expectancy (DFLE), an indicator derived from mortality and information on impairments or disabilities, which uses the life expectancy table technique, represents an important expansion of the concept of life expectancy, since it enables a differentiation to be made between the number of years lived free from any type of impairment or disability and the number of years lived with at least one impairment or disability.

Table 13. Percentage Distribution of Employed People Aged 10 Years and over, in the Reference Week, by Type of Disability and Occupation Groups of the Primary Job, Brazil, 2000.

Occupation Groups of Primary Job	Percentage Distribution of Employed People Aged 10 Years and over in the Reference Week (%)								
	Total (1) (2)	Type of Disability							
		At least one type of disability	Permanent mental disability	Physical impairment		Unable, with some or great permanent difficulty seeing	Unable, with some or great permanent difficulty hearing	Unable, with some or great permanent difficulty hearing, working or climbing stairs	No disability
				Permanent tetraplegia, paraplegia or hemiplegia	Total or partial absence of limb (3)				
Total	100.0	100.0	100.0	100.0	100.0	100.0	100.0	100.0	100.0
Armed Forces	0.9	0.4	0.6	0.2	0.2	0.4	0.5	0.3	0.9
Legislator, senior officials and managers	4.3	3.3	3.4	3.4	3.7	3.2	3.4	2.8	4.4
Professionals	5.8	4.1	4.7	5.2	3.1	3.9	3.7	3.3	6.1
Technicians and associate professionals	7.8	6.1	5.8	6.9	5.0	6.1	5.5	5.0	8.1
Clerks	8.2	5.2	5.6	8.9	4.8	5.1	4.1	4.2	8.7
Service workers and shop and market sales workers	29.6	31.5	29.2	33.1	23.8	32.0	28.0	35.8	29.3
Skilled, agricultural and fishery workers	17.6	24.7	26.5	19.5	24.1	25.9	26.3	26.8	16.4
Craft and related trade workers	22.1	21.0	20.1	18.7	30.4	19.9	24.3	18.5	22.3
Maintenance and repairs	2.4	2.1	2.2	2.4	3.3	1.9	2.7	1.7	2.4
Occupation not classified by field	1.4	1.5	1.9	1.9	1.6	1.6	1.5	1.6	1.4

Source: IBGE, 2000 Census.

(1) People with more than one type of disability were counted only once. (2) Including people without answer to the questions on disability.

Table 14. Percentage Distribution of Employed People Aged 10 Years and over, in the Reference Week, by Type of Disability, Sex and Nominal Monthly Income Classes of All Jobs – Brazil, 2000.

Sex and Nominal Monthly Income Classes of All Jobs (Minimum Salary)	Percentage Distribution of Employed People Aged 10 Years and over in the Reference Week (%)							
	Total (1) (2)	Type of Disability						
		At least one type of disability	Permanent mental disability	Physical impairment	Unable, with some or great permanent difficulty seeing	Unable, with some or great permanent difficulty hearing	Unable, with some or great permanent difficulty hearing, walking or climbing stairs	No disability
Total	100.0	100.0	100.0	100.0	100.0	100.0	100.0	100.0
Without income	7.6	10.6	12.8	8.1	11.1	11.3	12.6	7.2
Unit 1	23.3	29.5	31.3	27.4	30.4	28.2	33.4	22.4
More than 1 to 5	50.8	45.9	41.6	50.4	45.2	45.5	43.1	51.6
More than 5 to 20	15.7	12.2	12.2	12.5	11.6	13.1	9.7	16.3
More than 20	2.5	1.8	2.1	1.7	1.7	2.0	1.3	2.6
Male	100.0	100.0	100.0	100.0	100.0	100.0	100.0	100.0
Without income	7.0	8.9	12.6	7.5	9.2	9.8	10.8	6.7
Unit 1	20.2	25.7	30.5	25.8	26.4	24.6	29.9	19.3
More than 1 to 5	52.0	48.5	41.7	51.6	48.1	47.7	45.5	52.6
More than 5 to 20	17.6	14.6	12.8	13.3	14.0	15.4	12.0	18.1
More than 20	3.1	2.4	2.5	1.9	2.3	2.5	1.8	3.3
Female	100.0	100.0	100.0	100.0	100.0	100.0	100.0	100.0
Without income	8.7	13.3	13.3	10.9	13.9	14.8	15.1	8.0
Unit 1	28.5	35.7	33.1	34.2	36.4	36.9	38.0	27.3
More than 1 to 5	48.8	41.8	41.3	45.0	41.0	40.0	39.8	49.9
More than 5 to 20	12.6	8.3	10.9	9.1	8.0	7.4	6.6	13.3
More than 20	1.4	0.9	1.4	0.8	0.8	0.8	0.6	1.5

Source: IBGE, 2000 Census.
(1) People with more than one type of disability were counted only once. (2) Including people without answer to the questions on disability.

The most normal method to construct the indicator is the method proposed by Sullivan (1971) and consists of using the functions l_x and ${}_nL_x$, the number of survivors at age x and the number of years lived between the ages of x and $x+n$ of a life expectancy table previously constructed for the population studied.

The DFLE indicators were generated for the total for the Country and Regions, based on (Table 15) prevalence of at least one of the disabilities investigated.

The set of results shows that in Brazil in the year 2000 the DFLE was 54 years, representing 79% of the total of 68.6 years to be lived. The differential between the sexes of 3.8 years was lower than the 7.8 years of difference in life expectancy at birth. The regional variation in the DFLE however was more expressive than that observed when considering only mortality. The extreme values of DFLE were observed in the Southeast (56.7 years) and the Northeast (49.5 years), with a difference of 7.2 years.

Establishing the parameters of the country as a criterion, it can be observed that the Southern and Southeastern regions had, in the case of both sexes, superior life expectancies and disability-free life expectancies than those of the total for the country.

In the Northeastern region the indicators were extremely low, while in the Northern region the life expectancy at birth was near the country value, however the DFLE was significantly lower than the national average, showing a lower ratio between the years lived free of disability and the total life expectancy.

The regional variation in the DFLE was higher in females, by approximately 9 years, the variation in males being only 5.6 years. Both extremes occurred also in the Southeast and Northeast regions (Graph 12).

The regions with the greatest socioeconomic development, the Southeast, South and Midwest, show the best indicators, the Southeast being the region where around 81% of the years to be lived are free from any of the disabilities investigated.

Although the Northeast region shows high mortality and inferior socioeconomic indicators, the proportion of years free from disability of the number of years to be lived was lower than that observed in the Northern region, whose mortality was in an intermediate position. This reversal in behavior can be explained by a higher mortality rate of disabled people in the Northeast.

The ratio between the disability-free life expectancy and the normal life expectancy, which represents the proportion of the total number of years to be lived without disabilities, was greater for males than females in all regions. The higher male mortality rate influences these differences, since it leads to a large contingent of elderly females with disability.

Table 15. Life Expectancy (LE) and Disability-Free Life Expectancy (DFLE) by Sex – Brazil and Regions, 2000, All Disabilities.

Regions	Life Expectancy at Birth (LE)			Disability-Free Life Expectancy at Birth (DFLE)			Ratio DFLE/LE			Gender Diference in Ratio DFLE/LE
	Both Sex	Male	Female	Both Sex	Male	Female	Both Sex	Male	Female	
Brazil	68.6	64.8	72.6	54.0	52.1	55.9	78.7	80.4	77.0	3.4
North	68.5	65.6	71.7	50.4	49.5	51.4	73.6	75.5	71.6	3.9
Northeast	65.8	62.7	68.9	49.5	48.5	50.5	75.3	77.4	73.4	4.0
Southeast	69.6	65.1	74.3	56.7	54.1	59.3	81.4	83.1	79.8	3.2
South	71.0	67.3	75.0	56.2	54.1	58.3	79.1	80.4	77.8	2.7
Central West	69.4	66.2	73.0	54.0	52.7	55.4	77.8	79.5	75.9	3.6

Note: For building DFLE indicator were used the life tables from IBGE.
Source: IBGE, Research Directory

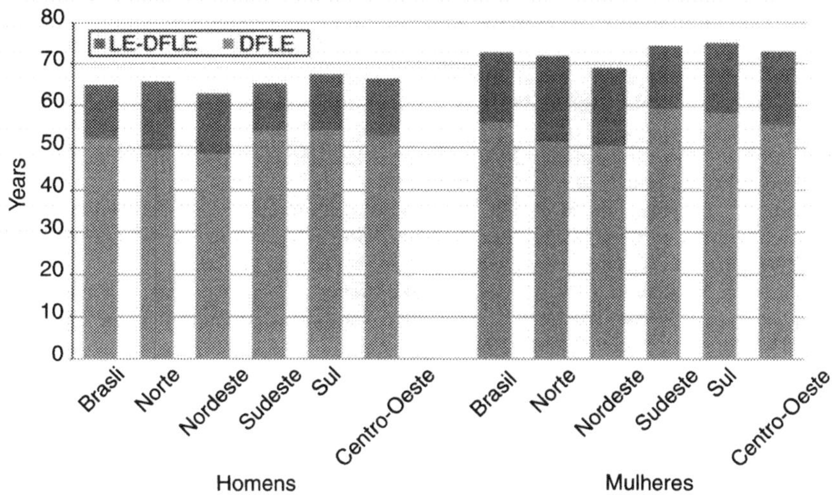

Graph 12. Life Expectancy (LE) and Disability-Free Life Expectancy (DFLE), by Sex and Regions, Brazil 2000. *Source:* IBGE, 2000 Census.

NOTES

1. For this study people with severe disabilities were considered to be those that declared themselves incapable or with great difficulty in seeing, hearing or walking. Therefore people that declared they have some difficulty in those domains mentioned were excluded.

ACKNOWLEDGMENTS

The author is grateful to Marcia Martins, Jacqueline Manhães, Eliane Xavier, Ana Paula Miceli, Andréa Barbosa, Andréa Diniz, Andréa Borges e Rodrigo Lemes who collaborated with important comments, calculations, tables and graphs.

REFERENCES

Brazil, (1989) Law No. 7.853 dated October 24, 1989. Regulates the support for disability, their social integration, the national coordination department for the integration of disability (CORDE), institutes the jurisdictional guardianship of the collective or diffuse interests of these individuals, regulates the action of the Public Prosecutor, defines crimes and introduces other measures. Official Gazette of the Federal Republic of Brazil, Brasília, DF, October 25, 1989. Section I, p. 1920.

Hernández-Licona, G. (2001). *Disability and the labor market: Data gaps and needs in Latin America and the Caribbean.* Washington, DC: Inter-American Development Bank, Sustainable Development, Social Programs Division.

IBGE, (2000). Life Tables (Brazil). IBGE Web site <http://www.ibge.gov.br>. Access January 21, 2003.

IBGE, (2003). Censo Demográfico 2000: Características gerais da população – resultados da amostra (pp. 60–82). Rio de Janeiro: IBGE.

Mbogoni, M., & Synneborn, M. (2003). General disability measures in developing countries – relationship to purposes for measurement. Paper presented at the 2nd meeting of the Washington City Group on disability statistics. Ottawa, Canada.

Montes, A., & Massiah, E. (2001). *Disability data: Survey and methods issues in Latin America and the Caribbean.* Washington, DC: Inter-American Development Bank, Sustainable Development, Social Programs Division.

Porter, G. L. (2001). *Disability and education: Toward an inclusive approach.* Washington, DC: Inter-American Development Bank, Sustainable Development, Social Programs Division.

Sullivan, D. F. (1971). *A single index of mortality and morbidity.* HSMSA Health Reports (Vol. 86, pp. 347–354), apr. <http://www.statcan.ca/start.html>. Access January 21, 2003.

World Health Organization (2001). International Classification of Functioning. Disability and Health – ICF, Geneva.

FURTHER READING

Mbogoni, M. (2002). Disability census questions: The perspective of developing countries. Paper presented at the 1st meeting of the Washington City Group on disability statistics. Washington, DC, United Nations.

Mbogoni, M., & Me, A. (2002). Revising the United Nations census recommendations on disability. Paper presented at the 1st meeting of the Washington City Group on disability statistics. Washington, DC, United Nations.

United Nations. (1998). *Principles and recommendations for population and housing censuses.* New York: United Nations Statistical Papers, Series M, n. 67/ver. 1.

United Nations. (2001). *Guidelines and principles for the development of disability statistics.* New York: United Nations Statistics on Special Population Groups, Series Y, n. 10.

United Nations. (2002). *Report of the Washington City Group on disability measurement.* Washington, DC: United Nations Statistical Commission.

MONITORING PEOPLE WITH DISABILITIES: THE ITALIAN EXPERIENCE

Roberta Crialesi and Elena De Palma

ABSTRACT

The aim of this article is to present the project "Information System on Disability", carried out by ISTAT (Italian National Statistics Institute). The background context affecting its implementation is described, in terms of both the policies and the main information sources on disability available in Italy. The paper does not attempt to develop a new theoretical explanation of disability, but underlines the steps and actions that must be taken, and problems that must be overcome in building a statistical information system on disability able to satisfy the information needs of diverse users.

INTRODUCTION

Disability is once more at the center of policy discussions in Italy as well as in all European Union countries[1] and beyond. The growing limitations of public resources and the downsizing of welfare programs make it necessary to readdress all topics related to supporting individuals, including those

International Views on Disability Measures: Moving Toward Comparative Measurement
Research in Social Science and Disability, Volume 4, 159–176

ISSN: 1479-3547/doi:10.1016/S1479-3547(05)04010-8

related to disability, and to find new strategies. Social integration is considered as a key issue for this population, thus monitoring life conditions of people with disabilities is a crucial part of fighting discrimination and promoting equal participation in society.

In Italy, the approach to disability issues and policies addressing the rights and needs of people with disabilities has undergone continuous change since 1992. There are two laws relevant to this paper: Law #104 – "Assistance, Social Integration and Rights of Handicapped Persons"[2] – which was adopted by Parliament in 1992, and Law #162 – "Modifications to Law n. 104" – adopted in 1998. The first law (#104/92) is a milestone in Italian disability legislation, because it addresses different aspects of disability through a holistic approach. This law initiated an integration process among policies and services and activated a number of interventions in various social contexts to overcome barriers preventing people with disabilities from achieving equal opportunities and full integration into social life. The law promoted preventive services and early diagnosis, treatment, assistance and rehabilitation, scholastic integration and professional training, work placement and social participation.

The second law (#162/98) established further services regarding specific disability-related issues. It also underlined the importance of statistical data for policymakers, and promoted a stronger dialog amongst all bodies (public institutions and private organizations) involved in promoting integration of people with disabilities. In particular, the law states that the Minister of Welfare must promote surveys on disability and organize a national conference every three years. The main goal of the conference is to evaluate social and health policies and identify new steps to be taken in enforcing the rights of people with disabilities. The conference results are given to Parliament for further discussion on improving legislation.

Policymakers need up-to-date information on different issues related to disability, so that they can monitor the efficacy of current policies and plan new strategies for interventions. The increase in demand for policy-relevant statistics has resulted in a proliferation of data sources, which use different concepts, definitions, methods and units for data collection. This creates an apparent or real contradiction among data, which often gives an incomplete picture of the situation, causing disorientation to data users (Egidi, 2000). In these conditions, statistical data cannot fully support policy-related issues. More efforts should therefore be made to improve and implement a new statistical information system to establish regular and systematic data collections and reports.

This paper presents the "Disability Information System" project, being executed by the Italian National Statistics Institute (ISTAT). Its main goal is to build a statistical information system on disability, based on a comprehensive set of indicators aimed at monitoring implemented policies. This paper outlines the steps and actions taken in the project's implementation, its challenges and its main products.

THE "DISABILITY INFORMATION SYSTEM" PROJECT

At the end of 1999, following implementation of Law #162/98, the Minister of Welfare entrusted ISTAT with the development of the "Information System on Disability" project.

The following five main steps were taken to develop the project:

- Review and analysis of information needs for policymakers and other potential data users, thus allowing better identification of the objectives to be pursued through the indicators system;
- Identification of data sources on disability in the country;
- Development of a conceptual framework, laying out aspects of disability which need to be known and monitored;
- Creation of the architectural design for the information system, and identification of the most appropriate formats and practices to make data available to users;
- Implementation of specific actions to overcome the current lack of available information related to disability issues and to fully exploit local data sources.

First Step: Review and Analysis of Information Needs for Potential Data Users

The goal here was to identify the data requirements for the main users of an information data system on disability. Statistical information on people with disabilities is in fact of interest not only to policymakers, but also, for example, for prevention and rehabilitation program managers; managers of health, social, educational, recreational and transportation services; academic and research organizations; associations of persons with disabilities and their families; insurance companies; producers of technologies for people with disabilities; and the general public and mass media. The kind of information needed and the way in which it is utilized is clearly connected to the role and functions fulfilled by the users including policy planning and allocation of economic resources; implementation of prevention and rehabilitation programs; development of services and evaluation of policies and services; monitoring of government actions; and academic research and information diffusion. Moreover, while the national policy needs clear, precise, summarized information on the population, which is not too specific but gives enough information on the relevant points, regional policymakers need more disaggregated and specific data allowing detailed understanding of the situation in their area and for more specific policy purposes. For instance in Italy, Public Administrations have a strong central position in the welfare sector while Regions, Provinces and Municipalities are the local authorities responsible for social and health policy planning at the local level. Regions deal mainly with planning and resource allocation (and so require general indicators at the regional level), while Provinces and Municipalities are responsible for actual implementation of the plans (and thus need more specific, program-oriented indicators such as those that document local demand for and supply of specific services for the person with disability).

To fully understand these information needs, meetings were held with policymakers and other representatives from various types of data users. This led to a greater and more detailed comprehension of their requirements and how they could be satisfied.

Basic questions such as: "How many people with disabilities are there in the population?" "What kinds of disability do people in the population have? What is the prevalence of the various disabilities?" were of interest to all data users. However, much more is needed to plan and monitor policies and services provided, and to integrate them among several sectors (health, education, employment, etc.) (UN, 1996). In general, to target services appropriately, it is important to know how the prevalence of disability varies by age group, gender and geographical areas; the economical condition of people with disabilities; specific needs and special appliances or aids required and other environmental barriers to be overcome in all contexts (home, school, workplace, transportation, recreation services, etc.).

With regard to other data users, epidemiologists are more interested in the causes of functional limitations and the process which leads to a disabling condition. They thus require both disaggregated and longitudinal data. In contrast, associations of persons with disabilities need qualitative data in addition to quantitative, especially on life conditions, in order to promote respect for the human rights of people with disabilities, lobby for better legislation and monitor its implementation. Finally, citizens in general want to know if social policies have achieved their goals, and if allocated resources have been fully and effectively utilized. They are thus more interested in informative indicators, able to describe if the life conditions of persons with disabilities have been improved.

Second Step: Identification of Data Sources on Disability in Italy

Identification of the information sources available in Italy was necessary for the construction of a more accurate picture of the various data producers, aspects of disability investigated/surveyed and main characteristics of the available data (ISTAT, 2000). In Italy, as in other countries, data sources on persons with disabilities may be grouped under two general headings: administrative records or registers and population surveys.

The administrative sources were the major source of information on disability until the 1980s. This information was usually collected for non-statistical reasons, mainly related to administrative activities, as required for a particular program or service for disabled persons meeting specific inclusion criteria. Various administrative records and registers have been used to generate information on disability at a national level. These include specific target group populations such as:

- people drawing invalidity[3] pensions and allowances awarded (National Social Security Institute, INPS);
- workers with disability due to an industrial accident or disease (National Institute for Industrial Accident Insurance, INAIL);
- people with disabilities drawing an assistance pension or an allowance for assistance from a third party (Ministry of Interior);
- pupils with visual, aural or psycho–physical impairments in ordinary education (Ministry of Education);
- children with a mental, physical or sensory impairment in special education (Ministry of Education);
- unemployed persons with disabilities (Ministry of Labor);
- people with sports-related disabilities (SPORTASS-CONI).

To this list must be added the Information System of the National Health Services (Ministry of Health), the Driving Licenses Archive (Ministry of Infrastructures and Transportation), and the Survey of the Italian Sports Federation for people with disabilities.

With respect to population surveys, in 1980 ISTAT carried out the first Health Interview Survey, investigating for the first time at national level the topic of permanent invalidity. This provided a new opportunity to analyze the social demographic profile of persons with permanent invalidities. The survey took into account only some of the disabilities contained in the International Classification of Impairments, Disabilities and Handicaps (ICIDH – WHO, 1980) (persons with visual impairments and a mixture of hearing and speech impairments and movement disability), and therefore underestimated the number of people with permanent disabilities. Over the years, other health surveys were conducted in 1986–1987, 1990 and 1994; new questions were included to investigate in greater detail the theme of personal autonomy in the functions of everyday life.

ISTAT has been committed to facilitating communication among data sources and having them interact with the targets and resources. Toward this end, a new social survey system on households called "Multi-Purpose Household Surveys System" has been developed. Its structure is simple: a yearly survey, forming a basic informative picture on the quality of life and daily behavior (including health-related aspects) of Italian citizens, which is periodically supplemented with questionnaires on specific aspects. For the first time the theme of disability is thoroughly examined by a methodology reasonably faithful to WHO indications and recommendations on ICIDH actuation. The Multi-Purpose Household Surveys System annually supplies information on the integration of people with disabilities, through the survey component "Aspects of daily life". Information on social networks is collected every five years with the in-depth survey "Households, social subjects and conditions of childhood".

The Health Interview Survey (HIS), carried out every five years in the framework of the Multi-Purpose Household Surveys System, is of great importance. The latest HIS (1999–2000) was the first to be performed in collaboration with the Ministry of Health and Regional Administrations which gave financial support to the sample expansion, for the purpose of allowing estimations on health and lifestyles at a sub-regional level (60,000 households, 150,000 persons). For the first time, some aspects of well-being (based on the SF12 measure), social autonomy (using ADL and IADL)[4] and extra-residential services (home care, day-hospital and so on) were studied in more depth. These aspects play a strategic role in interpreting the social and health conditions of people with disabilities.

At local (regional/provincial) level other data sources also provide useful information on their reference area in their specific context of data gathering. However, often these cannot be utilized in building the national picture, due to the different definitions and measures used. These include institutional data sources such as Regional Social and Health Service Authorities, local health authorities and hospitals, Job Centers, and non-institutional sources such as associations of people with disabilities, non-profit organizations and insurance companies.

Briefly, in Italy there is an ample range of data sources on disability, but they are discontinuous in both their cover and the definitions of disability used. In addition information, when it exists, is very often not accessible to all potential users, as it remains within the institutions which produce it.

Third Step: Build a Conceptual Framework

To select an appropriate and comprehensive indicator set, it is essential to build a conceptual framework as a reference tool (ISTAT, 2000; Egidi & Buratta, 1999). This also allows a "consensus" to be reached among the different actors (mainly data producers) in the information system, to encourage data exchange and permit construction of an information base for the indicator system.

The conceptual framework is based on three perspectives of the data user: (1) specific areas of policy interest; (2) specific target population groups; and (3) specific causes of disabilities.

The "specific area of policy interest" refers to the various thematic areas identified on the basis of national legislation, with main reference to the previously mentioned Law #104/92 ("Assistance, Social Integration and Rights of Handicapped Persons"), and the principal European and international guidelines. Priority areas include Health, Education, Employment, Social Participation, Access and Mobility and the Social Security System. Some of the broader actions and services included in the Law (#104/92) are: *Health*, the law specifies concrete actions to be taken on early prevention, care and rehabilitation and stresses the need to provide integrated health and social services which "maximize the abilities of each person"; *Education*, the law proposes specific tools such as the "individual education plan" (performed in collaboration with the family) and the "individual functional profile", to be drawn up by a multidisciplinary team, and aimed at monitoring a dynamic process to maximize individual school results; *Employment*, the law now specifies that "residual working capability" be assessed, with the aim of fostering better target insertion in accordance with the company's needs. With the legislation related to *Social participation*, the law emphasizes the importance of integration of people with disabilities and proposes services which ensure this (family fostering and placement in socio-rehabilitative and educational day-centers, community accommodation and family houses). It also prohibits any form of discrimination by public service providers in their dealings with people with disabilities. Finally, with *Access and Mobility*, the law ratifies interventions aimed at removing obstacles to performing daily, sporting, recreational and tourist activities and at improving interpersonal communication and access to information. For the *Social Security System*, the law identifies better criteria and standards in providing economic support.

The perspective "specific target population groups" is intended to directly focus attention on those most at risk of social exclusion and on those for whom specific measures of social intervention are aimed. For example, people with a severe reduction in autonomy need special attention, as do women, children and elderly people with disabilities and people with disabilities in institutions. One particular unit of analysis is the Household, which can provide information on the met and unmet needs of families taking care of a member with disabilities. This issue is particularly important in Italy, where the family is the main source of support and mediation between individual needs, especially of its weakest members, and the resources of society.

The perspective specific "causes of disabilities" aims to capture critical events and phases in life in which problems may arise which lead to disability, and which should therefore be monitored. In this area, the indicators would permit evaluation of the association of a specific pathology or debilitating event with health services and planned prevention policies. The causes of disability of interest are: congenital malformation, disability caused by an accident (domestic, traffic or industrial) and disability caused by illness.

The principal dimensions to be monitored were identified in line with these three user perspectives, with the aim of constructing a comprehensive set of indicators to cover all disabilities for which sustainable data collection is available. The appendix presents a non-exhaustive list of dimensions for which indicators important in describing people with disabilities have already been implemented.

Fourth Step: Design the Information System Architecture

A consultation process was carried out with national and local institutions producing or gathering data on disability. Best practices in developing and managing of other information systems on social, health and disability issues were identified and seminars were organized for more detailed comprehension of their objectives, structure and functioning. These activities allowed identification of other data sources and creation of a collaborative network among data producers.

The "core" of the information system architecture is the "indicators system".

Taking into account that statistical information is a useful tool for several types of users with different information needs and expertise in using statistical data, the system architecture includes other products such as a Metadata system and a Data warehouse. These were developed to support easy and friendly access to the data presented through the indicators system. In addition, a web site was created to allow free access to all data on disability available in Italy.

Fifth Step: Implementation of Specific Actions to Overcome the Disability Information Gap

The last step of the project was to understand what actions could be taken to build a coherent information system on disability, by improving existing data sources and setting up new ones where necessary. Since the beginning of the project, it has been clear that the major problem was the lack of effectiveness of existing data and lack of coordination among various databases and records, causing disorientation in its users and depriving decision makers of an essential tool. It was also clear that a great amount of data at local administrative level was underutilized as a data source (ISTAT, 2000). Comparison of the conceptual framework for the selection of indicators and data available for them highlighted the importance of the information gap. For all these reasons, surveys on the registers and data available from various local institutional bodies and on certification data were carried out. An in-depth survey on people with disabilities was also performed, as a first step in investigating other disability-related issues and providing a wider picture of the life conditions and needs of persons with disabilities and their families.

To summarize, two principal work lines were established to implement the "Disability Information System" project: (a) a brief period of analytical activity, to evaluate existing data and make them easily available to all users through the information system; and (b) a long period aimed mainly at improving existing statistical sources, promoting coordinated information flow and producing data on specific topics previously less investigated.

The following pages describe in detail the system's architecture and various products from the project.

PRODUCTS OF THE DISABILITY INFORMATION SYSTEM

The Web Site

The web site www.disabilitaincifre.it was planned as a tool for diffusion of statistical information, facilitating data accessibility and reinforcing the relationship between data producers and users. The site allows interrogation of the implemented indicator system through a predefined query system, and gives access to all important information on the correct use of indicators. It is also possible to request the construction of personalized tables through the data warehouse. The web site also allows access to results reached through realization of other products from the project, such as surveys performed, and offers more information about disability, which may be useful to a wider public. It is accessible to disabled persons, respecting in fact the CAST (Center for Applied Special Technology) rules on accessibility.

The Disability Indicators System

The indicators system, as already noted, is the core of the whole "disability information system". The conceptual framework, based on three perspectives of the data user (area of policy interest, target population, causes of disability), provided the main reference for its construction. However, it was necessary to reconcile the theoretical approach with the actual availability of the data essential for its construction. The system contains not only specific indicators directly connected to the characteristics of the policies to be monitored nationwide, but also those capable of comparison with the European situation, in line with the data harmonization process currently in progress in the European Statistical System (Eurostat, 2002; ISTAT, 2001a). Almost 400 indicators, selected on the basis of their policy relevance and validity, are currently included in the system. They are broken down by sex, age and geographical area and in some cases time series are also included.

The indicators system still face many shortcomings such as comparability, reliability, poor relationships among indicators inadequate or inappropriate differentials. Some aspects of disability are insufficiently covered and there is a great difference in level of coverage among different areas. Data scarcity significantly limited the development of the user perspectives "target population group" and "causes of disability". This lack is due to the fact that more appropriate measurement tools are needed, especially to understand the problems of childhood disability and mental disability (NCHS, 2002; ISTAT, 2000; ISTAT, 2001b; EUROSTAT, 2002); with regard to the perspective of the target population group, while no document exists which determines which and to what extent various pathologies are disabling. In addition, this user approach requires the availability of longitudinal data on the same individual, in order to monitor the evolution of conditions over time. This type of data is not yet available. Overcoming these limits and widening the thematic contents according to the three user perspectives remain as goals at which future efforts will be directed.

Metadata System

The Metadata system is one of the most important communication tools between data producers and users, particularly when an information system is based on multiple data sources. Detailed information on data sources, definitions, classifications and methodologies used in both data collection and indicator calculation is crucial in supporting the integration and harmonization of statistical information. The Metadata consists of Explanation of Indicators, Description of Data Sources, and Glossary. The *Explanation of Indicators* provides information necessary for correct data interpretation such as rationale and relevance of the indicators, type of data sources (population surveys, administrative records), definition of disability used and year(s) of reference. It appears automatically before every table when consulting the site. The *Data Sources* section describes in detail all sources from which data were used. For each, the following parameters are described: type of survey, definition of disability used, unit of data collection, unit of analysis, frequency of data collection, institution responsible for the survey, survey design, type of sample, available and published territorial detail, data quality and variables surveyed. The *Glossary* contains all "technical" terms used, and is particularly useful for users unfamiliar with statistical terminology or themes of disability.

All information on the Metadata system is available both by consulting the area created specifically within the site and through following links during its navigation.

Data Warehouse

The data warehouse is useful for more expert users and those with a precise objective or in search of specific data. It consists of an interrogation system allowing data extraction from the various information sources and construction of personalized tables in accordance with available data (criteria are defined to ensure that laws on privacy are respected). The user is guided to choose and relate classification variables and analysis units to obtain the table desired.

The main analysis units are currently: Families, Individuals, Services and Assistance, Schools, Sports Societies, Accidents, Pensions and Benefits and Special Driving Licenses. The main classification variables are Health Assistance, Economic Conditions, Culture and Information, Work, Social Assistance and Protection, Health, School and Education, Socio-demographics, Lifestyles and Geographical Area. Both the analysis units and the classification variables will be expanded as other data become available. To fully exploit all available regional data, the data warehouse has been planned as an open system that can be supplemented with autonomously gathered data from regional sources. This will not only complete the picture of disability in Italy but also provide a work tool for policymakers and social workers interested in a specific geographical area.

Registers Available at Local Level Containing Information on Disability

At the local level, there are many archives and databases on disability, which need to be taken into account for a complete and detailed picture of disability in Italy.

To this end a survey was conducted using two questionnaires sent to the following main bodies: Regions, Local Health Authorities, Provinces, Prefectures and Education Offices. The first questionnaire asked information on the Body's typology and possession of data relating to disability issues. Where a positive response was given, further information was requested on the field of data gathered (diagnosis, social services, rehabilitation services, tourism, mobility, employment, etc.) in the previous two years. The second questionnaire surveyed in detail the characteristics of each information data source indicated in the first questionnaire, such as the elementary unit (type of services) on which information was studied or recorded, method of data acquisition (ad hoc questionnaire, disability assessment reports) and the characteristics gathered in the enquiry model (variables studied). Also requested was the classification of disability used (ICIDH, ICIDH2,[5] other international or local classification) and the measurement tool for severity of disability. A notable difference was found in the classifications used, making data comparison from these sources more difficult. The questionnaire also contained questions regarding quality data, ways in which the information is used; level and typology of distribution of data gathered from these sources. A great deal of information was found to be held in a non-electronic form, which is a major obstacle in the reorganizing data of exchange.

The information gathered from this survey was organized to create a Register, which is available on the project's web site. This is quickly and easily accessible to a wide variety of users through use of a search engine by key word (e.g. type of body and field in which information is collected; geographical level). Selection of the research criteria (key words) leads to a summary of information gathered by these data sources. To allow its continuous update, the Register has also been planned as an open system, allowing the Bodies to update their situation as new information becomes available.

Pilot Survey on Disability Certification

In Italy, an important information source on disability is Local Health Authority certification data. However, there are currently several obstacles to its use: the certificates themselves are issued by specific evaluation commissions whose composition varies with the type of certificate (e.g. certifications of disability and its severity, certifications for school placements of disabled pupils or for workplace insertion) and different definitions and classifications of disability are used. In addition, most certification is registered on paper only, inhibiting its detailed analysis. To overcome these obstacles, an electronic certification form has been designed with the collaboration of Regional Authority and Local Health Authority managers and experts. This model (in electronic version or on paper for those without computer access) includes a core set of information to be filled in for each certificate issued by the Local Health Authority. Primary fields included in the model are: identification of the Local Health Authority, date of certification, reason for certification, results of the evaluation commission, tax code of the person requiring the certificate, citizenship, place of birth and residence, family situation, qualifications and employment conditions, type of disability (ICIDH, ICF) and type of pathology (ICD 10). The tax code number allows identification of all certification issued for the same person, while the national law on privacy is respected through use of specific procedures. This model will be tested in a pilot study together with the methods of data transmission, processing and use. Its nationwide implementation will finally allow registration of all people legally recognized as having a disability. This continuously updated archive can also be used as a reference base for the realization of surveys to investigate in greater depth aspects of disability.

Survey on Persons with Disabilities

The current data available at national level on disability does not give a complete picture on some important issues such as the needs of persons with disabilities and their families, satisfaction with services supplied, formal and informal help networks and level of social integration. Also missing is information which would allow monitoring of changes in life and health conditions with time.

To respond to these needs an "ad hoc" survey is being prepared in collaboration with the Italian association of people with disabilities. The survey sample (4,000 individuals) includes people who declared a reduced autonomy (with or without assistive devices) in their activities of daily life in the 1999–2000 ISTAT survey "Conditions of Health and Recourse to Health Services". Apart from gathering socio-demographic information on the person with disabilities and his/her family, the survey particularly investigates the following aspects: typology of the reduction in autonomy, its cause and onset; activity limitations, process to reach diagnosis of the health problem; social and health services and interventions utilized, those which the individual would have liked but was unable to use and the reasons for this inability; scholastic and employment experiences and difficulties encountered, needs and responses obtained; mobility in cities and the countryside and social participation; presence or absence of architectural barriers of the building and inside the apartment where the person interviewed lives.

The results of this research will add significant new information for the planning of social policies, which will promote full participation of citizens with disabilities in various social contexts, and push for an improvement in the quality and characteristics of services for their benefit.

CONCLUDING REMARKS

Construction of a statistical information system on disability is a fundamental prerequisite in guiding policymakers in their choices as regards establishing priority scales, in performing a comparative evaluation of alternative intervention strategies, estimating costs and benefits of the different policies, and monitoring the effects on disability of interventions accomplished. However, an integrated and coordinated approach to the production of official statistics on disability has not yet been fully implemented in Italy. The implementation of the "Disability Information System" project presented here is an important step in this direction. It provides an indicators system as a reference tool for the policy decision-making process, built through consultation with policymakers, and it also organizes all available data within a single information system which is accessible through the Internet to all potential data users. In fact, it is extremely important not only to overcome fragmentized data production but also to improve accessibility and interpretability by developing an efficient data and metadata dissemination system on disability.

The problems faced in the project's development have demonstrated various weaknesses in the data production system, such as:

- *Lack of data sources covering all aspects of disability and living conditions of people with disabilities.* Various information gaps were discovered, especially with respect to disabled children, the mentally disabled, causes of disability and issues related to the role of environmental factors in activity limitation of people with disabilities in different contexts (school, work, social life, mobility). Longitudinal studies and data were also absent.
- *Lack of communication among information sources.* There are several institutional data sources, at both national and local level, but few have been planned as part of a single, integrated information system.
- *Lack of reliable and comparable data.* As we have seen, the diverse information sources (both administrative and non-administrative) utilize different conceptual paradigms and instruments to identify and collect information about disability.
- In fact, collection of information on people with disabilities is a complex task, which still requires great effort. It is necessary to promote a better and continued dialog between data producers and users as well as among data producers themselves; to link statistical surveys with administrative data and to reconcile different source figures and indicators. Furthermore, it is extremely important to establish regular and systematic collection; to adopt identical conceptual paradigms and common language, develop data collection on the above-mentioned aspects of disability and identify statistical reference instruments. The ICF (International Classification of Functioning, Disability and Health) represents an important resource in this area, as it offers a multi-perspective approach and proposes a common language applied in several fields (WHO, 2001). This will give great support to the integration and harmonization of data related to information system, registers and population surveys covering different aspects of disability.

NOTES

1. In addition to several official documents of the European Commission, in 2001 the Council of the European Union declared 2003 as the "European Year of People with disabilities". Eurostat has also promoted several research projects aimed at overcoming the lack of comprehensiveness, coherence, and comparability of data among European member states.

2. Article 3 of Law n. 104 of 1992 defines a "handicapped person" as someone who "has a physical, mental or sensorial disability, stable or progressive, which is the cause of difficulties in learning, relationships, or workplace integration and is of a degree to determine a process of social disadvantage or marginalization". The term "handicapped person" is no longer common. It has been replaced by "person with disabilities".

3. The condition of "civil invalidity" describes citizens affected by congenital or acquired disabilities causing at least a 33 percent reduction in working capability for those between 18 and 65, or a persistent difficulty in performing normal tasks and functions appropriate for the age group for those under 18 or over 65.

4. In the Health Interview Survey, a person with disabilities is considered as someone who has declared to have serious difficulty in performing at least one activity among the dimensions proposed by Activities of Daily Living (ADLs) scale (Katz, Ford, Moskowitz, Jackson, & Jaffe, 1963).

5. The survey was carried out before publication of the ICF.

REFERENCES

Council Decision of European Union of 3 December on the European Year of People with Disabilities 2003, 2001/903/CE.

Egidi, V. (2000). System of indicators for social policy. Presented at the 2000 Meeting of the Siena Group on Social Statistics, Maastricht, The Netherlands, 22–24 May 2000.

Egidi, V., & Buratta, V. (1999). The role of indicators in optimizing resources allocation. In: Essay (Ed), *9th Reves International Meeting Proceedings*, 11–13 December 1996, ISTAT publication.

EUROSTAT. (2002). *European Disability Measurement (EDM) Project*. Final report. Eurostat Working Paper – Population and social conditions 3/2002/E/N° 20, Luxembourg, European Commission.

ISTAT. (2000). *Progetto Sistema Informativo sull'Handicap. Fase 1: Studio di fattibilità*. Research Report, August 2000.

ISTAT. (2001a). *Indicators on integration of disabled persons into social life*. Report, June 2001.

ISTAT. (2001b). *Progetto Sistema Informativo sull'Handicap. Fase 2: Disegno concettuale del sistema informativo statistico*. Report, December 2001.

Katz, S., Ford, A. B., Moskowitz, R. W., Jackson, B. A., & Jaffe, M. W. (1963). Studies of illness in the aged. The Index of ADL: A standardized measure of biological and psychosocial function. *JAMA*, *185*(12), 914–919.

NCHS. (2002). Summary report of the first meeting in http://www.cdc.gov/nchs/citygroup.htm

United Nations. (1996). *Manual for the development of statistical information for disability programmes and policies*. New York: United Nations Publication.

WHO. (1980). *International classification of impairment, disabilities and handicaps*. Geneva: WHO.
WHO. (2001). *International classification of functioning, disability and health*. Geneva: WHO.

APPENDIX. MAIN DISABILITY DIMENSIONS INCLUDED IN THE INDICATORS SYSTEM OF "DISABILITY INFORMATION SYSTEM" PROJECT

Education and scholastic integration
Education level
Scholastic attendance
Scholastic success
State school support staff
Architectural barriers

Work and Employment
Employment level
Unemployment level
Working conditions
Assistance with work placement
Level of satisfaction

Health and Assistance
Health Status
Demand for health services (Home-based assistance, Rehabilitation, Hospitalization, Diagnosis, and Medical Consultations)
Health services supplied
Economic costs
Prevention

Social Participation
Community life (participation in formal and informal associations)
Recreation and leisure (including sport)
Holidays and Tourism
Religious participation
Political participation
Interpersonal relationships

Social Security System
Recipients of disability pensions or benefits
Social Security System Expenditures

Transportation services
Private transport
Public transport (use and level of satisfaction)

Households
Household context
Types of Households
Type of dwelling (including Architectural barriers)
Informal help and support network
Economic Resources

Accidents
Work-related accidents
Sporting accidents
Domestic accidents
Road accidents

SECTION III: METHODOLOGICAL ISSUES

TESTING A DISABILITY QUESTION FOR THE CENSUS☆

Ken Black

INTRODUCTION

In the International Classification of Functioning, Disability and Health (ICF) 2001, the World Health Organization (WHO) defines disability as: 'an umbrella term for impairments, activity limitations and participation restrictions. It denotes the negative aspects of the interaction between an individual (with a health condition) and that individual's contextual factors (environmental and personal factors)', with environmental factors including assistance from other people, from equipment and from formal sources. WHO previously defined disability, in the context of health experience, as "any restriction or lack (resulting from impairment) of ability to perform an action in the manner or within the range considered normal for a human being" (World Health Organization, 1980, p. 28).

The Australian Bureau of Statistics (ABS) has conducted regular Special Supplementary Surveys (SSS) since 1981 that provide detailed information on disability consistent with the original WHO definition, and also consistent with the new ICF. However, these surveys cannot provide estimates for

☆Views expressed in this paper are those of the authors and do not necessarily represent those of the Australian Bureau of Statistics. Where quoted or used, they should be attributed clearly to the authors.

International Views on Disability Measures: Moving Toward Comparative Measurement
Research in Social Science and Disability, Volume 4, 179–223

ISSN: 1479-3547/doi:10.1016/S1479-3547(05)04011-X

small geographical areas, the level at which disability and aged care services are often planned and delivered. Data also cannot be provided in relation to disability for relatively small population groups, e.g. Indigenous Australians or people from specific smaller non-Australian backgrounds. In Australia therefore, as in many countries, there is a demand for a disability question to be included on the national census.

The ABS criteria for the inclusion of a topic in the Census of Population and Housing include:

- that the topic is of major national importance;
- that there is a need for data on the topic for small groups of the population and for small geographical areas and
- the topic is suitable for collection via the census.

It is broadly agreed that the disability topic meets the first two criteria. However, there have been concerns about its ability to meet the third criterion because of the complex nature of defining and identifying disability, the limited space available on the census form and the method of form completion (self-enumeration by any household member).

This report discusses the methods and results of the testing conducted by the ABS in November 1997 and September 1998 for the 2001 Census of Population and Housing. It also provides background information on the history of collecting disability data in Australia and the rationale for testing a census question on disability.

History of Collecting Disability Data in Australia

The ABS has collected data on disability using both census and sample survey instruments. In response to the demand for handicap data, a question on handicap was included on the 1976 Census (see Appendix 1 for 1976 Census question). As shown in Table 1, almost 30% of the people who reported a handicap in the census reported no handicap in exactly the same question in the post-enumeration survey. Over 50% of those who were identified in the post-enumeration survey as having a handicap, did not identify themselves in the census handicap question. Further evaluation indicated that the data obtained from the handicap question were unreliable.

On the basis of these results, the disability and handicap topic was not included in later censuses.

In 1981, the International Year of Disabled Persons, the ABS conducted its first national survey on disability. Known as the Survey of Handicapped Persons, the collection identified people with a disability and addressed the

Table 1. Summary of Results from the 1976 Census[a].

Census handicap rate	3.5%
Survey handicap rate	5.9%
False-negative rate	
(Survey handicap, census no handicap) as a proportion of the survey handicap population	51.9%
False-positive rate	
(Survey no handicap, census handicap) as a proportion of the census handicap population	27.9%
Census to survey ratio	
(Census handicap population divided by the survey handicap population)	0.6

[a]For information on the meanings of these terms see – 'Census Testing' section.

nature and extent of their restrictions in activities of daily life, their use of aids and their ongoing need for assistance, receipt of assistance and unmet need.

The survey also provided information on the characteristics of people restricted by disability, including their living conditions, work, education and recreation.

These topics continued to be the focus in the following surveys, the Survey of Disabled and Aged Persons in 1988 and the Survey of Disability, Ageing and Carers (SDAC) in 1993 and 1998 (disability criteria and related definitions for the 1998 survey can be found in Appendix 2). As information needs developed over time, in line with government policies and social attitudes, the population groups of interest expanded to include older people and carers and some new topics emerged while others were seen as no longer relevant.

Since the 1993 SDAC, a shorter set of disability questions has been included as a module in other ABS surveys. These surveys include:

- Household Expenditure Survey 1993/94 and 1997/98;
- Time Use Survey 1992 and 1997;
- 1992 Survey of Training and Education;
- 1997 Education and Training Experience Survey;
- the longitudinal Survey of Employment and Unemployment Patterns (1994–95, 1995–96, 1996–97); and
- the General Social Survey and Indigenous General Social Survey (2002).

Demand for Inclusion of Disability in the Census

The ABS national disability surveys provide a considerable amount of data on disability. The main limitation from a user perspective is that this information cannot be produced for small geographic areas, or small population groups from a sample survey.

Support services such as accommodation, in-home support, activity programs; living skills training and employment services for people with a disability and home care or help for older people are often organised and delivered at a local level. The demand for small area data is likely to rise as there is increasing emphasis being placed on regional planning of community services. Consequently, there is a high level of demand for the census to provide information on the prevalence of disability in the Australian population that can be used in conjunction with the more detailed survey data.

To compensate for lack of census data, small area predictors have been modelled using disability survey data and census population information. However, these do not reflect concentrations of people with disabilities because of special service provisions or risk factors in an area. In addition, for adequate and sensitive delivery of personal services, information is needed at the small area level about people of different ages and diverse backgrounds.

In particular there has been a call for more detailed information on the Indigenous disability population, which has not been successfully collected in existing disability or Indigenous collections, although for the first time the ABS is including a disability module within both the General Social Survey (GSS), and Indigenous General Social Survey (IGSS) to be enumerated in 2002.

In 1993, the disability survey used a sample size of about 17,000 households. Given the proportion of Indigenous people in the population and a sample of this size, there should have been approximately 900 Indigenous respondents including about 175 with a disability. In fact, because of the difficulties of disability identification in this population and the problem with Indigenous coverage, the numbers were considerably smaller than these expectations. The 1993 survey included 660 people who were Indigenous of whom 59 were identified as having a disability. Successful collection of information on disability in the census would provide more useful data on the Indigenous disability population (no Indigenous identifier was included in the 1998 disability survey, nor is it planned for 2003).

There is public interest in the inclusion of disability on the census. In the round of submissions regarding the content of the 1996 Census, 48 submissions out of around 280 submissions were received supporting the inclusion of disability. Despite the number of submissions received, the ABS initially did not intend to include disability on the 1996 Census.

This decision was made in the light of the poor quality of the data collected in other censuses, e.g. in the United States of America, Canada, Great

Britain and New Zealand as well as in the 1976 Australian Census. However, following further discussions on Census content and strong lobbying by a number of users, this decision was reconsidered.

It was finally agreed that the ABS should test a suitable question on disability in the 1993 census test. The quality of the data obtained would be measured by comparing the results with data collected through a personal interview follow-up survey (using the screening questions from the Disability, Ageing and Carers survey). Two disability questions relating to the need for assistance because of disability, for possible inclusion in the census, were tested in Melbourne in November 1993. These questions did not provide reliable results compatible with the follow-up survey. Because of the poor quality of data obtained during testing, disability was not included as a topic in the 1996 Census.

Following the 1996 Census, eight letters from government ministers were received regarding the exclusion of disability in 1996 and asking that it be considered in future censuses. In the last round of consultations about the content of the 2001 Census, disability attracted the largest number of submissions (31), with strong support for disability status to be collected in subsequent censuses.

Considerable testing and revision of census disability questions for the 2001 Census again failed to produce reliable results that were consistent with the follow-up survey using the criteria of the SDAC. As a result, it was recommended that disability not be included as a topic in the 2001 Census.

CENSUS TESTING

The 2001 Census disability question testing used a different approach to previous tests, based on questions relating to difficulties experienced with everyday activities. Following discussions with the Census Consultative Group on Disability, testing was undertaken through a series of focus groups and two census tests conducted in November 1997 and September 1998 (for details on the 1998 questions see Appendices 3 and 4).

Conduct of Census Disability Tests

1. A sample of census districts (a geographical area usually containing about 250 dwellings, designed for the purposes of a population census data collection) is selected. These districts might be chosen to increase the likely capture of the population of interest.

2. Census test forms are distributed to all households in the selected census districts.
3. The forms are completed by at least one member of the household for the whole household on the census test night.
4. Census test forms are collected.
5. Follow-up information (follow-up survey) is collected via personal interview from a responsible adult in respect of all persons in the household included on the census form (this may not be completed by the same person who completed the census test form).
6. Census form results and the personal interview results are then compared.

Indicators Used to Evaluate Census Disability Tests

The primary measures the ABS uses to decide whether the disability questions tested are suitable for use in the census are how well and how consistently the populations identified as having or not having a disability match the populations that would be identified by the SDAC. Accordingly, the follow-up questionnaires were based on the initial screening questions in the SDAC (SSS16 in 1993 and SSS28 in 1998). These screen questions provide the benchmark.

The following constitutes a disability identification match:

Census response positive ↔ interview response positive
Census response negative ↔ interview response negative.

Two types of mismatch are identified:

Census response negative → interview response positive = false negative
Census response positive → interview response negative = false positive.

Identified on the Census	Identified in the Follow-Up Survey	
	Disability	No disability
Disability	Matched disability (matched positive)	False positive
No disability	False negative	Matched non-disability (matched negative)

Table 2 provides definitions of the indicators used to evaluate the census disability tests. Some indicators are expressed as a proportion of the survey

Table 2. Indicators and Results – The Measures Used to Evaluate the Census Disability Tests.

Indicator	Definition	Formula	Purpose of the Indicators
Matched disability (or matched positive)	People who were recorded with a disability in both the census and survey		To show how well the census questions capture the populations identified with a disability in the follow-up survey
Matched disability rate	Persons who were identified with a disability in both the census and survey *as a proportion of the survey disability population*	(Matched disability/survey disability) × 100	100% represents a perfect match Rate of 80% considered acceptable
Matched non-disability (or matched negative)	People who were recorded without a disability in both the census and survey		To show how well the census questions capture the non-disability populations identified in the follow-up survey
Matched non-disability rate	Persons who were identified without a disability in both the census and survey *as a proportion of the survey non-disability population*	(Matched non-disability/survey non-disability) × 100	100% represents a perfect match Rate of 80% considered acceptable
False positive	Persons who were identified with a disability in the census but not the follow-up survey		To show the accuracy of response of people answering the question in the census – those who incorrectly identified themselves with a disability

Table 2. *(Continued)*

Indicator	Definition	Formula	Purpose of the Indicators
False-positive rate	Persons who were identified with a disability in the census but not the follow-up survey *as a proportion of the census disability population*	(False positive/census disability) × 100	0% represents a perfect match Rate of 20% considered acceptable
False negative	Person who were identified in the follow-up survey with disability but not in the census		To show the accuracy of response of people answering the question in the census – those who failed to correctly identify themselves with a disability
False-negative rate	Persons who were identified in the follow-up survey with disability but not in the census *as a proportion of the survey disability population*	(False negative/survey disability) × 100	0% represents a perfect match Rate of 20% considered acceptable
Census disability	Total people in the census population identified with a disability	(Matched disability + false positives)	To show the percentage of the total population who were identified by the census questions with a disability
Census disability rate	Total people in the census population identified with a disability by the census question *as a proportion of the total population*	(Census disability/total) × 100	Census disability rate = survey disability rate represents a perfect match

Survey disability	Total people in the survey population identified with disability	(Matched disability + false negatives)	To show the percentage of people who were identified by the survey questions with a disability
Survey disability rate	Total people identified in the follow-up survey with a disability *as a proportion of the total population*	(Survey disability/total) × 100	
Overall match (total matched in the total population)	Total number of respondents matched (matched disability plus matched no disability) *as a proportion of total population*	(Matched disability + matched non-disability)/total × 100	To show how accurately the census responses matched with the survey responses for the whole population 100% represents a perfect match
Census to survey ratio	Census disability population *as a proportion of survey disability population*	Census disability population/survey disability population□	To show the consistency between the census disability rate and the survey disability rate overall and for small population groups and geographical areas 1.0 represents a perfect match

or census disability populations, while others are a percentage of the total population for ease of understanding the overall effect.

Criteria for Evaluating the Census Tests

Three different sets of criteria were selected to evaluate the census test results and determine if the results were good enough to consider inclusion in the census:

1. High rate of matched positives identified on the census test and the follow-up survey:
   - 80% of the survey identified population also identified on the census
   - 80% of the census identified population also identified on the survey.
2. A close relationship between the census disability rate and the follow-up survey disability rate (census to survey ratio = 1 would be a perfect result).
3. A consistent census to survey ratio for small areas and small populations.

To produce an acceptable result and for the disability questions to be considered for inclusion in the census, one of the following combinations of the above criteria had to be met:

- Criterion 1 + Criterion 3: consider collecting disability in the census, may not be published to the public; or
- Criterion 2 + Criterion 3: consider collecting disability in the census, may not be published to the public; or *ideally*
- Criterion 1 + Criterion 2 + Criterion 3: collect disability in the census, publish results.

NOVEMBER 1997 CENSUS TEST FOR THE 2001 CENSUS OF POPULATION AND HOUSING

As agreed with the Census Consultative Group on Disability, a different approach for the 2001 Census was taken from that used in 1993 for the 1996 Census. For the 2001 Census the criterion for disability was difficulty in performing a range of activities rather than the need for assistance, as in the 1993 Census test, which identified a narrower group. After focus groups were conducted, a special census disability test was conducted in Victoria in November 1997. Collection districts were selected from Melbourne and regional centres in areas known to have a higher proportion of people with disabilities. The filter question established a 'health' context for the activity question.

Aim

The aim of the November 1997 Census test was to test the feasibility of a question focussing on difficulties with activities for possible inclusion in the 2001 Census of Population and Housing.

Pre-testing of the Questions Using Focus Groups

Leading up to the November 1997 Census test, focus groups were commissioned to investigate the wording of the Census disability questions. Focus groups were designed to see how well the questions worked for relevant sub-populations, particularly whether these groups understood the disability questions and understood what was meant by disability.

First Wave of Focus Group Testing

The first round of focus group testing for the 2001 Census disability questions took place in August 1997. A total of 59 people were given both sets of questions.

The focus groups consisted of:

- two general groups of people aged 15–59 years;
- people aged 60 years and over;
- people with an intellectual disability – with carers;
- people with an intellectual disability – independent; and
- people with a psychiatric disability.

Two versions were tested. The first question of version 1 asked if the persons had a physical or mental illness, health problem or disability that had lasted 6 months or more. The second question asked if this long-term condition caused difficulty with or stopped them from doing a number of activities: physical activities, communicating in own language, learning, understanding or remembering things, any other difficulties or none of the above.

In version 2, the first question asked if the person found it impossible or difficult to do a number of activities: everyday activities; communication or socialising; learning, understanding or remembering things; any activity that people the same age could usually do; or none of the above. The second question asked what caused the difficulty: disability, long-term health condition (lasting 6 months or more), short-term health condition, age or other – please specify.

The results from the focus groups were not promising, with version 2 being more prone to misinterpretation. Problems with correct answering of the questions were prominent for those with an intellectual disability, some older people and those where English was their second language. However, the results of this testing provided some useful recommendations to improve the census disability questions.

The recommendations were:

- simplify version 1 so that only disability and health condition are identified and reverse their order;
- separate some of the activities so that less words and fewer activities are combined;
- change ordering of reasons for difficulty from least important to most important (short-term illness first through to disability last);
- add 'difficulty with language' to reasons for difficulty – use this to filter difficulty because of English as a second language from difficulty because of a disability; and
- exclude the word 'impossible' and use the word 'difficulty'.

Second Wave of Focus Group Testing

The second round of focus group testing was undertaken in September/October 1997. A total of 65 people were involved. Focus groups were undertaken for:

- indigenous people;
- people with intellectual and physical disabilities;
- people with mental illnesses;
- aged people living in an institutional care setting;
- carers of people with disabilities;
- carers of aged people; and
- general population.

Two more versions (versions 3 and 4) of the census disability questions were tested and all participants completed both versions, with some completing version 3 first and others completing version 4 first. Version 3 of the census disability questions placed the question on activity limitation first followed by the more direct question on disability while version 4 reversed the order. Participants also completed a private questionnaire to help assess their answers (the physically and intellectually disabled people were not required to complete this questionnaire), followed by an open-ended discussion on the strengths and weaknesses of the disability questions.

The focus groups found that both variants of the questions worked successfully. Version 3 was found to be a more reliable measure with participants preferring this question because it allowed the possibility of explaining more about the disability or health condition. Although the Indigenous population preferred version 4 of the questions, because it appeared to them to be less difficult to answer, the results for the Indigenous population were more successful on version 3.

The recommendation was that version 3 should be adapted in the light of the focus group testing findings for the November 1997 Census test.

Details of the 1997 Census Test

In the 2 weeks from 21 November to 5 December 1997, census forms were delivered to around 2,600 households, which were to be completed on 26 November 1997. When the census form was collected, an interviewer conducted a follow-up survey in respect of all the persons in the household. There was a response rate of 78%, which resulted in 5,406 respondents in the final sample.

Results of the 1997 Test

Rate of Match

The disability questions tested in the November 1997 Census test performed better than those tested in 1993 with a match of 52% between the census and survey disability populations. There were, however, unacceptable levels of false negatives (48%) and to a lesser extent false positives (17%) (Table 3).

Conclusion

The disability question results from the November 1997 Census test did not satisfy the requirements for a successful test. The matched disability rate of 52% and the similar results for both the census and the follow-up survey within collection districts that varied across districts provided some hope that the questions were measuring an identifiable subset of disability. However, the high level of false negatives (48%) and the false positives (17%) were of concern.

This test had performed better than the previous attempts to measure disability in a census question, and some of the results were encouraging

Table 3. Summary of Results from the November 1997 Test.

Census disability rate	14.5%
Survey disability rate	23.1%
Matched disability rate (matched census disability as a proportion of the survey disability population)	52.0%
Matched non-disability rate (matched census non-disability as a proportion of the survey non-disability population)	96.7%
Matched disability (% of total)	12.0%
Matched non-disability (% of total)	74.4%
Total matched in test population (% of total)	86.4%
False-negative rate (survey disability, census no disability) as a proportion of the survey disability population	48.0%
False-positive rate (survey no disability, census disability) as a proportion of the census disability population	17.4%
Census to survey ratio (census handicap population divided by the survey handicap population)	0.6

enough to justify a further test. The main problems were the high rate of false negatives and the lack of consistency for small population groups. The Census Disability Advisory Group suggested that a scaled response might cut back the false negatives and assist in identifying a more useful population, on the grounds that:

- respondents would feel more comfortable answering 'a little' than 'yes'; and
- the 'a lot' response might indicate a population with greater support need.

There was a further possibility that the census might be measuring an identifiable sub-group of the survey disability population.

SEPTEMBER 1998 CENSUS TEST FOR THE 2001 CENSUS OF POPULATION AND HOUSING

Following the recommendations from the evaluation of the 1997 disability census test, the modified questions were tested in Adelaide in September 1998.

Aim

The second test was part of a full-scale census test of 20 collection districts. The aim of the disability part of this second test was to:

- evaluate whether a scale (none/a little/a lot), rather than a yes/no response, would decrease false-negative responses and improve the match with disability status measured in the follow-up survey;
- measure whether disability identified by the census questions, or by the 'a lot' census responses, had a stable relationship with an identifiable subset of the disability population (as measured in the follow-up survey); and
- further test consistency for small population groups and small areas.

Details of the Test

The September 1998 Test used a split sample to test two sets of questions. The two sets were:

- Form type 4 – respondents were asked to indicate 'no' or 'yes' to whether they had difficulty with a range of several functions (e.g. hearing, living independently). The question was very similar to that used in the November 1997 test.
- Form type 5 – respondents were asked to indicate whether they had 'none', 'a little' or 'a lot' of difficulty with the same seven functions (scaled response) (see Appendices 3 and 4 for the September 1998 form type 4 and form type 5 disability questions).

Response

Census responses were received from 4,536 dwellings of the 5,425 dwellings approached for the September census test (84% response rate). A total of 10,573 people completed the disability questions on the census forms. A follow-up survey was conducted with around half of the households where a census form had been collected.

Follow-up interviews began once census collectors provided lists of the dwellings with completed census forms. Analysis was based on the population (5,695 people) that completed the follow-up survey. The people in households where the follow-up survey was conducted had a similar demographic profile to the census test sample with a slight bias to households with older people, children and people working part-time or not in the labour force, where there was a greater likelihood of making contact.

Composition

The difference between the age structure and the ethnic composition in the September 1998 test (conducted in South Australia) and the November 1997 Census test (conducted in Victoria), reflected differences in the population structure of the two states. A higher proportion of the 1998 South Australian test population was aged 60 years and over – 25.7%, compared with 19.0% in the 1997 Victorian test population. There was a correspondingly lower proportion of those aged 0–14 years in the 1998 test population.

The South Australian test had a higher proportion of people born in Europe and a lower proportion of people born in Asia, the Middle East and North Africa and other countries. The proportion of males and females was similar on both the 1997 and 1998 tests.

Results of September 1998 Test

A range of different criteria for constructing disability was examined for both the census and the follow-up survey. The best result obtained was where the follow-up survey disability definition was based on that used in the SDAC, 1998 (the person had one or more restricting impairments from the survey screening question set, see Appendix 2 for restricting impairment list under 'disability'), and the most straightforward census disability definition where:

Disability is identified if:

- any response in Q18 is 'yes' (form type 4), 'a little' or 'a lot' (form type 5) and in Q19 is 'disability';
- any response in Q18 is 'yes' (form type 4), 'a little' or 'a lot' (form type 5) and in Q19 is 'long-term condition';
- any response in Q18 is 'yes' (form type 4), 'a little' or 'a lot' (form type 5) and in Q19 is 'age' and the person is aged 60 years or more;
- there are zero 'yes', 'a little' or ' a lot' responses in Q18 but in Q19 is 'disability';
- response to Q18B 'hearing' is 'yes' (form type 4), 'a little' or 'a lot' (form type 5) and the person was born in Australia or an English-speaking country and is aged 3 or more and
- response to Q18C 'learning, understanding or remembering things' is 'yes' (form type 4), 'a little' or 'a lot' (form type 5) and the person is aged 9 or more.

All results in this report for the 1998 test are based on these definitions.

Form type 4 contained a 'yes' response and form type 5 the responses 'a little' and 'a lot'. All the data included in this section are based on this census/survey match definition.

As suggested, the scaled response reduced the false negatives and led to a much higher matched disability rate (66%) (see Table 4). However, this was at the cost of a greatly increased false-positive rate.

Table 4. Summary of Results, September 1998.

	Form Type 4 (Yes/no response)	Form Type 5 (Scaled response)
Census disability rate	15.0%	22.4%
Survey disability rate	19.9%	21.7%
Matched disability rate (matched census disability as a proportion of the survey disability population)	52.1%	65.9%
Matched non-disability rate (matched census non-disability as a proportion of the survey non-disability population)	94.2%	89.7%
Matched disability (% of total)	10.4%	14.3%
Matched non-disability (% of total)	75.5%	70.2%
Total matched in test population (% of total)	85.8%	84.5%
False-negative rate (survey disability, census no disability) as a proportion of the survey disability population	47.9%	34.1%
False-positive rate (survey no disability, census disability) as a proportion of the census disability population	30.9%	36.0%
Census to survey ratio (census handicap population divided by the survey handicap population)	0.8	1.0

A closer correspondence between the census disability population and an identified subset of the survey population in consequence did not eventuate. Hopes for a consistent census to survey ratio were disappointed.

False Positives

The false-positive rates in 1998 (31% for form type 4 and 36% for form type 5) were much higher than those in the November 1997 test (17%).

However, analysis of the false-positive population does give some indications of factors contributing to the increase in false positives. The contributing factors are:

- The introduction of a scale in form type 5 made it easier to give false-positive responses. Responses of 'a little' or 'a lot' were available. Where people were not sure whether the level of difficulty they have is high enough for a positive response, it was easier to answer 'a little' than an absolute 'yes'.
- A false-positive response was more likely to be given for the older population and there was a higher proportion of older people in the 1998 South Australian Census test population (Table 5). For form type 4, almost 10% of those aged 60 years and over had a false-positive response

Table 5. False Positives by Age and Sex, November 1997 and September 1998.

	November 1997		September 1998			
			Form type 4		Form type 5	
	False positives	All persons	False positives	All persons	False positives	All persons
	(%)	(%)	(%)	(%)	(%)	(%)
Age						
0–14 years	11.2	21.4	7.6	16.7	5.2	16.1
15–59 years	53.9	60.7	42.0	59.2	39.8	56.7
60 years and over	34.9	18.0	50.4	24.2	55.0	27.3
All persons	100.0	100.0	100.0	100.0	100.0	100.0
Sex						
Males	52.0	48.2	51.1	47.5	51.9	48.2
Females	48.0	51.8	48.9	52.5	48.1	51.8
All persons	100.0	100.0	100.0	100.0	100.0	100.0

compared to 2% and 3% for 0–14 years and 15–59 years, respectively. For form type 5, the rate was 16% of those aged 60 years and over, compared to 3% for 0–14 years and 6% for 15–59 years.

- The percentage of people who were classified as false positive or false negative in the census test varied between birthplaces. For form type 4, those from other European countries had a higher percentage of false positives, false negatives and matched positives. These higher percentages may be age-related rather than strictly related to birthplace. For form type 5, other European countries had a higher percentage of false negatives, those born in Northeast, Southeast and Southern Asian countries had a higher percentage of false positives and those born in other countries had a higher percentage of false negatives.
- A small number of people may have misinterpreted the census question on difficulties experienced and indicated all the areas where they had no difficulties, particularly for form type 4. Approximately 9% of the false positives in form type 4 (yes/no) had ticked all responses to the 'difficulties' question and then indicated in the subsequent question that they had no difficulties. This figure was about 2% for the form type 5 (none/a little/a lot).

False positives were high on form type 4 where it was reported that they did not speak English at all (23%) and also where the proficiency in English

Table 6. Self-Reported Proficiency in English by False Positives, September 1998.

	Form Type 4 (%)	Form Type 5 (%)
Self-reported proficiency in English		
English only	4.0	8.7
Very well	3.9	3.8
Well	9.3	7.0
Not well	7.7	12.0
Not at all	23.1	5.6
Not answered	13.6	6.1
All persons	4.6	8.1

question was not answered (14%) (Table 6). For form type 5, false positives were higher where it was reported that English was not spoken well (12%).

Around four in ten (38%) of the false positives had reported a disability or long-term condition as the reason for experiencing difficulty. A similar proportion (38%) gave age as the reason for their difficulties. Most of the latter were aged 60 years or over. These are valid responses for disability and were found in comparable proportions among the matched positives.

It is difficult to establish a good rate of matched disability results using the census questions and an independent follow-up survey up to a month later. False positives may result from:

- a different person responding to the follow-up survey from the person(s) completing the census;
- varying responses at different times;
- varying response to self-enumeration of the census test and interview in the follow-up survey and
- the different angle of approach in the survey (a wide group of restricting impairments) from the difficulty with specified activities used in the census questions.

False Negatives

Compared with the November 1997 false-negative results (48%), false negatives from the September 1998 test were similar (48%) for form type 4 and lower (34%) for form type 5. Factors may have been:

- The census test disability questions in form type 5 were designed to reduce the number of false negatives.

- There was a relationship between age and the recording of false negatives on the census test in 1998. For form type 5, 12% of the respondents aged 60 years and over gave false negatives, while 3% of respondents aged 0–14 years, and 7% of respondents aged 15–59 years gave false negatives.
- Most of the people with false negatives in the September 1998 test (87%) indicated no difficulties in the first census disability question, and also stated 'no difficulty' or did not respond to the second question, despite a positive response to the follow-up survey. The majority of the remaining few false negatives had reported a difficulty or reason for a difficulty in the census, but did not fully meet the census disability criteria (see Appendix 2). Possible changes to the census criteria to capture the remaining cases were identified but discarded, as they would have increased the false positives.

CONSISTENCY FOR SMALL AREAS AND GROUPS

The scaled response of form type 5 showed greater consistency between the census and survey disability rates across census collection districts (CDs) than the yes/no option of form type 4. The greater consistency of ratio in form type 5 was not good enough, however, to warrant inclusion as a disability component in the 2001 Census, when the high rates of false negatives and false positives are taken into consideration. These results suggest that a scaled format of questions on disability within the census has some potential to identify the proportion of people with a disability within, and their distribution, across small areas. Such results might be useful in allocating funds to areas according to need, but the high variation in the results means that such a measure would not allow any useful identification of the characteristics of individuals who have been identified as having a disability.

Based on these results, it is recommended that any further testing on the inclusion of a disability component on the census should use a scaled approach rather than the yes/no option.

At the recommendation of the Census Advisory Group, further analysis was carried out on small geographic areas for a different age split (0–64 years and 65 years and over) to determine if better age-related small-area disability data could be produced. The ages correspond better to the scope of government support policy, disability services under 65 and aged care services at 65 and over.

The analysis showed that the poor census to survey ratios found for small-area data were less attributable to the 65 and over age group that had a better result within census districts than for those aged 0–64 years, with a matched disability rate of 80% or more in 11 of the 20 census districts and 70% or more in a further five. These results, however, continued to vary across the census districts with some areas producing poorer matches and some with very good matches having poorer ratios because of a high level of false positives.

The younger age group had much poorer matched disability rates, with high rates of both false positives and negatives. Overall, both groups had a census to survey ratio within 10% of the perfect one, masking a level of variation between districts. The older group, however, had a more concentrated mode, with 10 of the 20 districts having a ratio within 10% of 1, while in the younger group only 6 out of 20 were within this range.

One conclusion that can be drawn from this is that the census disability question may better identify the proportion of older people with a disability than those under 65 years in small areas. It is more important however, for a census disability question to correctly identify the geographical location of people in younger age groups with a disability for disability services planning and funding. There are much higher rates of disability among those in the older age groups, and therefore the concentration of older people in geographical regions can be used as a proxy to identify where funding and services for older people with disabilities are to be distributed. Any further work should focus on improving the measurement of younger people with disabilities across small geographical areas.

Small Population Groups

- Form type 4 under-represented the disability rate for all age groups. Form type 5 was a better indicator, particularly for the age group 0–14 years. Although the rates and the ratio suggest a good match, they mask a high rate of false positives and false negatives, which produce a much poorer match (Table 7).
- Consistent disability rates and ratios for different birthplace groups were not produced by either form type 4 or form type 5, although form type 5 was a better indicator for people from European and English-speaking countries (Table 7).
- The census disability questions do not provide consistent census to survey ratios across the small population groups of age, sex and birthplace. This was particularly predominant for birthplace. This, coupled with the high false positives and false negatives, suggest that the census disability questions do not provide an adequate measure of disability. However, the scaled response of form type 5 performed better than the yes/no approach of form type 4 (Table 7).

Table 7. Population Groups: Disability Rates, September 1998.

	Form Type 4 (Yes/No)				Form Type 5 (Scaled Response)			
	Census disability rate	Survey disability rate	Matched disability rate	Census to survey ratio	Census disability rate	Survey disability rate	Matched disability rate	Census to survey ratio
	(%)	(%)	(%)	ratio	(%)	(%)	(%)	ratio
Age								
0–14 years	5.7	6.4	56.7	0.9	5.9	5.9	55.6	1.0
15–59 years	9.4	14.3	42.7	0.7	12.8	13.7	52.0	0.9
60 years and over	35.1	42.9	59.4	0.8	52.0	47.8	74.9	1.1
Sex								
Males	15.6	19.2	55.4	0.8	23.7	22.0	68.4	1.1
Females	14.4	20.5	49.3	0.7	21.1	21.5	63.4	1.0
Birthplace								
Australian, NZ, UK, North America, South Africa	12.9	17.4	53.3	0.7	20.2	19.1	64.9	1.1
Other European	27.0	33.9	50.7	0.8	35.5	37.0	69.5	1.0
Northeast, Southeast and Southern Asian	11.9	9.5	75.0	1.3	23.3	18.6	62.5	1.3
Middle East and North Africa	9.1	9.1	100.0	1.0	20.0	20.0	100.0	1.0
Other countries	16.1	16.1	25.0	1.0	20.8	29.2	50.0	0.7
Not answered	12.1	33.3	27.3	0.4	18.8	22.9	63.6	0.8
All persons	15.0	19.9	52.1	0.8	22.4	21.7	65.9	1.0

Further analysis was carried out for disaggregation of age groups using the under 65 and the 65 and over split. The aim of this analysis was to test whether a disability question in the census may be reliable for certain age groups of special interest. Age was broken down into 0–14 years, 15–49 years, 50–64 years and 65 and over. The 50–64 years group is of particular interest, as this is a group where male participation in the labour force has been declining for a number of years and where the number of both males and females on the Disability Support Pension peaks (Table 8).

As expected, because of the association of disability with ageing, for both form type 4 and form type 5 the disability rate for 15–49 years (9% census disability rate for form type 5) was lower than for 15–59 years (13% census disability rate for form type 5) and the 65 and over age group had a disability rate higher (56% census disability rate for form type 5) than the 60 and over age group (52% census disability rate for form type 5) (Table 7).

On the more stable form type 5, the 50–64 age group performed better than the younger groups with a better match rate, lower false positives and negatives and a perfect ratio. The 65 and over age group, however, had a much higher matched disability rate (Table 8).

The following tables indicate how well the two form types capture the sub-groups of the disability population identified in the follow-up survey. These tables do not take false-positive responses into account.

Table 8. Variant Age Groups: Disability Rates, September 1998.

	Matched Disability Rate	False Positives	False Negatives	Census Disability Rate	Survey Disability Rate	Census to Survey Ratio
	(%)	(%)	(%)	(%)	(%)	(%)
Age groups						
Form type 4						
0–14	56.7	37.0	43.3	5.7	6.4	0.9
15–49	36.7	44.0	63.3	6.4	9.8	0.7
50–64	47.9	29.1	52.1	20.8	30.8	0.7
65 and over	62.7	25.6	37.3	39.3	46.6	0.8
All persons	52.1	30.9	47.9	15.0	19.9	0.8
Form type 5						
0–14	55.6	44.4	44.4	5.9	5.9	1.0
15–49	41.8	52.1	58.2	9.2	10.5	0.9
50–64	65.1	32.1	34.9	30.3	31.6	1.0
65 and over	78.2	31.5	21.8	55.9	48.9	1.1
All persons	65.9	36.0	34.1	22.4	21.7	1.0

Both form types were more able to identify a higher level of restriction; particularly keeping in mind that the level of restriction for these tests was not the initial basis for inclusion to the population of people with a disability. Form type 5 produced a consistently better match than form type 4.

- For those people who were classified as having a disability in the follow-up survey, a greater percentage was identified through the census questions for form type 5 (scaled response) than for form type 4 (yes/no response), 65.9% compared to 52.1% (Table 9).
- Only the disability types 'other long-term condition' and 'speech loss' produced a better result on form type 4 than form type 5, but the differences

Table 9. Level of Restriction: Matched Rate, September 1998.

	Form Type 4	Form Type 5
	Matched disability rate	Matched disability rate
	(%)	(%)
Populations		
Level of restriction		
Has severe/profound core activity restrictions	75.3	86.0
Has moderate core activity restrictions	56.0	71.7
Does not have moderate to profound core activity restriction	45.0	58.9
Has schooling or employment restrictions	62.3	71.2
Does not have schooling or employment restrictions[a]	25.5	39.5
Needs assistance with other everyday tasks	61.5	77.9
Does not need assistance with other everyday tasks but has difficulties	57.6	70.0
No difficulties in everyday activities[b]	40.0	54.9
All persons with disability on survey	52.1	65.9

[a]Only includes those persons aged between 5 and 64 years. All people outside of this age group were classified as not applicable.

[b]Only includes those persons aged 15 years and over. All people outside of this age group were classified as not applicable.

were small. Form type 5 is a better identifier of disability across most disability types.

- Hearing loss was well identified for people restricted by this impairment (79%) and those less restricted (81%); form type 5 also produced a good match rate for people with more serious psychiatric disability (91%), intellectual disability (80%) and some types of physical impairment.
- Most of the other impairment types on form type 5 had a match rate of over 70%. Only those with 'blackouts, fits, loss of consciousness', 'nervous/emotional condition', 'other long-term condition' and 'disfigurement/deformity' had a census to survey match under 70% (Table 10).

Table 10. Restricting Impairment: Matched Rate, September 1998.

	Form Type 4	Form Type 5
	Matched disability rate	Matched disability rate
	(%)	(%)
Populations		
Restricting impairment		
Has sight loss not corrected by glasses	51.0	72.5
Has hearing difficulties	72.5	78.5
Has loss of hearing: no aids or difficulty communicating	64.6	80.9
Has speech loss	73.7	71.4
Has difficulty breathing that restricts	65.3	81.0
Has chronic/recurring pain that restricts	59.2	73.6
Has blackouts, fits, loss of consciousness	36.0	57.7
Has difficulty learning/understanding	78.6	80.4
Has incomplete use of arms/fingers	60.7	77.2
Has difficulty gripping	62.0	73.0
Has incomplete use of legs/feet	69.9	82.9
Has a nervous/emotional condition	61.5	65.9
Restricted in physical activity	65.1	75.1
Has disfigurement/deformity	36.0	58.6
Needs help/supervision for mental illness	78.9	90.9
Has head injury, stroke or other brain damage	70.4	71.7
Receiving treatment for other long-term condition	56.8	72.0
Has other long-term condition	64.6	63.4
All persons with disability on survey	52.1	65.9

Matched Rates for Census Activity Restrictions

- The populations answering positively to each of the activity restrictions in census question 18 had very high matched disability rates, 90–100% in each form type (Table 11). This means that very few (up to 10%) of the people who had answered positively to a particular activity restriction but had not met all the criteria for a positive identification of disability in the census had been positively identified in the survey (i.e. they had been correctly disqualified from the census disability population).
- Most of the false negatives (see Table 6 – 48% in form type 4 and 34% in form type 5, respectively 10% and 7% of the total population responding to each form type) had either answered negatively or not answered the activity restriction question – they had positive identification in the survey, but had not provided a basis for positive identification in the census. The census question may be omitting an appropriate activity for identification.
- The census to survey ratio indicates the level of false positives in the population answering positively to activity restrictions. For the population with more severe restriction, those answering 'a lot', this over-count is within acceptable levels. The false-positive levels for form type 4 and for the 'a little' response for form type 5 are much higher, although the latter performs better.
- For the form type 5 population, the activities producing the highest over-count are 'hearing' and 'learning, understanding, remembering'. The inclusion of 'remembering' may lead to an over-response to difficulty in this activity, as it is common for many people to consider they have poor memories – further cognitive testing may be useful.

Conclusion

Form type 5 with the scaled response approach has shown a distinct improvement in decreasing false negatives compared with form type 4 and the earlier test. It performs well in capturing those with higher support needs, and has an improved capture rate for most impairments. It provides a very good census to survey ratio, and a reasonable consistency over small areas and some small populations. These good results, however, are offset by a higher false-positive rate and a still unacceptable rate of false negatives.

The analysis suggests some areas where further development and fine-tuning might improve the results, using form type 5:

- possible new activity, or modified presentation of existing ones, to better capture disability for the younger age groups;

Table 11. Activity Restriction (Census): Matched Disability Rate and Census to Survey Ratio, September 1998[a].

Census Question 18	Form Type 4		Form Type 5			
	Yes		A little		A lot	
	Matched disability rate[b]	Census to survey ratio[c]	Matched disability rate[b]	Census to survey ratio[c]	Matched disability rate[b]	Census to survey ratio[c]
	(%)	ratio	(%)	ratio	(%)	ratio
Activity restriction (using census test question)[d]						
Everyday activities i.e. eating, showering or dressing	98.4	1.6	93.3	1.1	97.9	1.1
Hearing	94.1	1.5	98.1	1.6	100.0	1.2
Learning, understanding, remembering	100.0	1.6	99.2	1.6	100.0	1.2
Reading or seeing even with glasses	89.6	1.5	89.9	1.4	94.3	1.2
Walking, kneeling or climbing stairs	94.4	1.3	94.9	1.4	96.2	1.1
Living independently	92.0	1.3	94.5	1.2	94.4	1.1

Table 11. *(Continued)*

Census Question 18	Form Type 4		Form Type 5			
	Yes		A little		A lot	
	Matched disability rate[b]	Census to survey ratio[c]	Matched disability rate[b]	Census to survey ratio[c]	Matched disability rate[b]	Census to survey ratio[c]
	(%)	ratio	(%)	ratio	(%)	ratio
Doing other things people of the same age usually do (i.e. working, studying, etc.)	95.3	1.3	97.3	1.3	95.0	1.1

[a]Includes only those who answered 'yes' to each activity restriction, excludes those answer 'no' or 'not stated'.
[b]Those identified with a disability in both the census and the survey.
[c]Census disability as a proportion of the survey disability population. With 1.0 being the best census to survey ratio.
[d]Question 18 in the census: for form type 4 'Mark YES or NO for each of the following: Does the person have difficulty …'; for form type 5 'How much difficulty does the person have in:' Each person may have more than one activity restriction.

- cognitive testing on the wording of questions producing high census to survey ratios:
  to identify which elements of the activity group prompt undue identification;
  to consider whether qualifying the identified elements might lower this effect;
- further cognitive testing work with immigrants from Asian countries to understand why their false-positive rates were high.

These attempts to match the results between the two census tests and survey results took no account of any response variance which might occur over time with repeated applications of either survey or census questions to the same set of respondents. No work has been done to quantify this variance. It is recommended that any future testing should include measures of response variance, for both the full survey and for any further questions developed for census testing.

ASSESSMENT OF CENSUS TESTS AGAINST EVALUATION CRITERIA

November 1997 Test

Criterion 1: *High rate* (*at least* 80%) *of matched positives identified on the census and the survey*. The results did not satisfy criterion 1.
Criterion 2: *Close relationship between census disability rate and survey disability rate*. The results did not satisfy criterion 2.
Criterion 3: *Consistent census to survey ratio for small areas and small populations*. The results did not satisfy criterion 3.

As no criteria were adequately met, none of the required combinations of criteria were satisfied. However, while the November 1997 Census test did not provide good enough results to warrant inclusion of disability questions in the 2001 Census, the results were promising enough to attempt another census test using modified questions.

September 1998 Test – Form Type 5

Criterion 1: *High rate* (*at least* 80%) *of matched positives identified on the census and the survey.*

- The overall matched disability rate was 66% for the survey disability population. This was higher than those found in form type 4 and in the 1997 test but does not meet the criterion of 80%.
- With a false-positive rate of 36%, 64% of the census disability population was correctly identified, not meeting the 80% criterion.
- The overall matched non-disability rate was 90%. This meets the criterion, but is lower than the matched non-disability rates for form type 4 and the 1997 Census test.
- The matched disability rates for collection districts for form type 5 ranged from 46% to 79%, with no areas achieving over the 80% range. However, the results across the collection districts were better than those found for form type 4 with most areas achieving around 60–70% matched disability rates.
- The matched disability rates for form type 5 were consistently better than those produced for both form type 4 and the 1997 test, but they were not consistent enough among the different population groups and small areas to justify inclusion in the 2001 Census. For some population groups, criterion 1 was met, while for other population groups this was not the case.

Criterion 2: *Close relationship between census disability rate and survey disability rate.*

- The overall census to survey ratio was 1.0. The disability rate for both the census and the survey was 22%, which also corresponds with the South Australian disability rate reported in the 1998 Survey of Disability, Ageing and Carers.

Form type 5 produced a much better result than Form type 4 and the 1997 Census test. Form type 5 met criterion 2.

Criterion 3: *Consistent census to survey ratio for small areas and small populations.*

- Census to survey ratios for collection districts ranged from 0.7 to 1.3, with the bulk close to the perfect result of 1.0. This may be considered acceptable.
- The census to survey ratios for small population groups varied between 0.7 and 1.3, with birthplace being less consistent than the other population groups. Age and sex produced more consistent census to survey ratios within 10% of the optimum result.
- For the 'a little' responses to the census activity restriction question the census to survey ratios varied between 1.1 and 1.6 showing over-counting in the census. For the 'a lot' responses to the activity restriction question

on the census, the census to survey ratio varied between 1.1 and 1.2, showing more consistent results than for the 'a little' responses. However, a large number of people identified with disability in the census had no or negative responses to the activity restriction questions.

Form type 5 produced more consistent census to survey ratios for small area data and small population groups than those found in form type 4 and the November 1997 Census test. However, although these ratios suggest that some consistent small-level data on disability can be collected using the census, they do not overall meet criterion 3 for inclusion in the 2001 Census. Future testing may suggest ways to improve these results to an acceptable level.

	Evaluation Criteria		
	Criterion 1	Criterion 2	Criterion 3
	(80% matched positives on census and survey)[a]	(Close relationship between census and survey disability rates)	(Consistent census to survey ratio for small population groups and areas)
Census test November 1997	X	X	X
September 1998 – form type 5[b]	X	✓	X

[a]This criterion plus one other criterion must be met.
[b]Criteria 1 and 3 were partially met for this census test.

The results for form type 5 in the September 1998 test produced better results than for form type 4 and the November 1997 Census test but did not meet the criteria for inclusion in the 2001 Census. The results provide some hope that scaled questions could be developed using the results from this test that may provide adequate results to include disability questions in a future census.

Attempting to find one or two questions that will produce a reliable measure of disability in a census is part of the wider problem of measuring disability. Disability covers a wide range of impairments, limitations and restrictions. The effects can vary for different people and even for the same person at different times. There can be a reluctance to identify with particular types of disability and this is likely to vary with time and also with the collection methodology. People may be more prepared to respond to an interviewer than to write information down on a form. The different results from form type 4 and form type 5 show the effect of an apparently simple change in response categories. Disability measures are sensitive to context – surrounding questions may encourage or discourage a positive response.

CONCLUSION AND CONSIDERATIONS FOR FURTHER WORK

Conclusions of Testing to Date

The ABS has made a considerable effort to design a census question set that would effectively measure disability in the census, particularly in the development period for the 2001 Census of Population and Housing. The results were not sufficiently successful to justify inclusion of the disability topic in the 2001 Census. The last variant tested, form type 5 with a scaled response, had problems with high false-positive response rates specifically associated with the use of a scale, but had improved results against a number of the assessment criteria.

The experiences of other countries indicate a similar lack of success in producing a good match between disability identification in a census and a follow-up survey, whether this be a repetition of the census question, or a more detailed survey question set. The best results reported have been from the UK census, measuring limiting long-term illness, although this concept differs from disability in the broader sense and could exclude people with a disability who do not regard themselves as having an 'illness'.

Whether to proceed with a census question where the validity of the results is doubtful becomes a matter of fitness for purpose. Where the primary purpose is to gain an enhanced sample for a survey, a quite high level of false-positive responses can be tolerated, as these can be corrected in the follow-up survey; a high level of false negatives would require a sampling of the 'no disability' population in the survey as well. Where the results are to be disseminated and used directly to inform policy and planning decisions for small areas and small populations, as would be the case in Australia, an assured high quality of census data is required.

A major difficulty the ABS has had with evaluating a census question is how well the results from a short question about activity limitation in a self-enumerated form could be expected to match with an interviewer-based detailed set of restricting impairment questions. The criteria to evaluate any further census tests are currently being considered.

While there are still substantial problems with the composition of the disability population identified in the census tests, analysis has pointed to areas where further work may produce more acceptable results. While this outcome cannot be guaranteed, and may not be probable, it justifies further testing and development.

The pressure for a disability question on the census remains strong; however, there are competing needs among potential users of census-based disability data. Information is needed at a small-area level to identify both the overall population of people with a disability, and the distribution of people with a disability likely to be receiving, or to be in need of service(s) related to disability and/or aged care. This latter population is identified in the SDAC via a complex set of questions on need for assistance and difficulty in a range of tasks within activity areas. The questions are asked of people already identified as having a disability via an initial set of screening questions.

Census testing so far has focussed on identifying the overall disability population in a way that was consistent and relatable to the full survey method. However, the 'target population' for government service funding/ provision is primarily the 'profound or severe' component identified in the ABS surveys (plus non-core activities for the Home and Community Care programs (HACC)), and at the end of the 2001 Census testing round, this population was identified as an alternative target population for future testing. This narrower population may be more easily and consistently identifiable in a census question, although this has not yet been confirmed by testing. The approach would involve identifying 'need for help or assistance' then sub-setting the identified population through a second question on the reason for the need. Responses of 'long-term disability/health condition' and 'old age' would contribute to the output population. To date in Australian testing, 'need for help or assistance' has only been used as a follow-on from an initial broader census question, hence the question may not have been asked of the appropriate population, with some components of the desired population having been already 'screened out' before the need for assistance could be identified.

RECOMMENDATIONS FOR 2006

The key issues for consideration by the 2006 Census Disability Advisory Committee are:

1. Determine the particular disability population to identify in the 2006 Census. There are two key options:

Option A. General disability population. To identify a broad disability population, similar to that identified in the SDAC. Starting from the 1998 form 5 approach, revisit in the light of questions used by Canada and New Zealand in their last census rounds. The Canadian and New Zealand question components and structures were similar to those tested in 1998 in Australia. Slight enhancements to the 1998 approach would enable a closer alignment to these other agency measures while retaining a close alignment to the SDAC concepts. Testing of the reasons for response differences (false positives and negatives) between the census and SDAC question sets should also be considered.

Option B. Profound/severe disability population. To identify the 'profound and severe' disability population, which is the key population of interest to the majority of service planners and funders in Australia. This would involve:

- asking an initial question about need/receipt of help or assistance within the core activity areas of personal care, mobility and communication;
- follow with a question on the reason for the need – e.g. 'disability or health condition lasting 6 months or more', 'old age', 'other'.

It could also be advantageous to include activity areas other than just the core, if responses can be separately identifiable. This could be particularly important for planning services such as HACC where the target population could be seen to be broader than that of disability program services. Appendix 6 is an example of the type of question, which could be further developed, with some activity areas other than just the core included.

Identifying 'need for assistance' in the general population, rather than as a follow-up relating to just the disability population, may result in output populations from the census and survey, which are not relatable. This would need to be carefully considered during testing if this approach was supported.

2. Determine the evaluation criteria to test the validity and reliability of the census disability question. It is important to determine how the disability population identified by the short census question relates to the full-survey disability populations and whether it is a useful, understandable and describable population suitable for small-area estimates.

3. Determine any other requirements that would assist in evaluating the census question. For example, consider testing the response variance of the

question both in terms of the census question(s) being tested, and of the full-survey question set.

The options recommended are for initial discussion purposes, and should not be seen as a final recommendation for the 2006 Census, particularly given the diverse needs of potential data users. These options, when considered with the results from the extensive testing so far, form the basis for discussion leading to agreement on a new approach for the 2006 development round.

POSTSCRIPT

Since the writing and presentation of this paper, there has been extensive ABS consultation about testing and evaluation of the proposed 'need for assistance' questions, now termed 'Core activity support needs'. This has resulted in the successful development of a set of questions suitable for inclusion in the 2006 Australian National Population Census. See Appendix 7 for the proposed questions. Details of testing conducted will be included in a future paper.

REFERENCES

World Health Organization. (1980). *International classification of impairments, disabilities, and handicaps: A manual of classification relating to the consequences of disease*. Geneva: World Health Organization.

FURTHER READING

Australian Bureau of Statistics. (1981). *Survey of handicapped persons, Australia, February – May 1981 (preliminary)*. Canberra: ABS Cat. no. 4342.0.

Australian Bureau of Statistics. (1982). *Handicapped persons, Australia, 1981*. Canberra: ABS Cat. no. 4343.0.

Australian Bureau of Statistics. (1990). *Disability and handicap, Australia, 1988*. Canberra: ABS Cat. no. 4120.0.

Australian Bureau of Statistics. (1993a). *Disability, ageing and carers: Summary of findings, Australia, 1993*. Canberra: ABS Cat. no. 4430.0.

Australian Bureau of Statistics. (1993b). *Disability, ageing and carers: User guide, 1993*. Canberra: ABS Cat. no. 4431.0.

Australian Bureau of Statistics. (1994a). *Disability census test: November 1993*. Census Working Paper 94/3.

Australian Bureau of Statistics. (1999a). *Disability, ageing and carers: Summary of findings, Australia, 1998*. Canberra: ABS Cat. no. 4430.0.
Australian Bureau of Statistics. (1999b). *Disability, ageing and carers: User guide, 1998*. Canberra: ABS Cat. no. 4431.0.
Australian Bureau of Statistics. (1999c). *Disability, ageing and carers: Summary tables, New South Wales, 1998*. Canberra: ABS Cat. no. 4430.1.040.001.
Australian Bureau of Statistics. (1999d). *Disability, ageing and carers: Summary tables, Victoria, 1998*. Canberra: ABS Cat. no. 4430.2.040.001.
Australian Bureau of Statistics. (1999e). *Disability, ageing and carers: Summary tables, Queensland, 1998*. Canberra: ABS Cat. no. 4430.3.040.001.
Australian Bureau of Statistics. (1999f). *Disability, ageing and carers: Summary tables, South Australia, 1998*. ABS: Canberra Cat. no. 4430.4.040.001.
Australian Bureau of Statistics. (1999g). *Disability, ageing and carers: Summary tables, Western Australia, 1998*. Canberra: ABS Cat. no. 4430.5.040.001.
Australian Bureau of Statistics. (1999h). *Disability, ageing and carers: Summary tables, Tasmania, 1998*. Canberra: ABS Cat. no. 4430.6.040.001.
Australian Bureau of Statistics. (1999i). *Disability, ageing and carers: Summary tables, Northern Territory, 1998*. Canberra: ABS Cat. no. 4430.7.040.001.
Australian Bureau of Statistics. (1999j). *Disability, ageing and carers: Summary tables, Australian Capital Territory, 1998*. Canberra: ABS Cat. no. 4430.8.040.001.
World Health Organization. (2001). *International classification of functioning, disability and health: ICF*. Geneva: World Health Organization.

APPENDIX 1. – 1976 CENSUS OF POPULATION AND HOUSING – CENSUS DISABILITY QUESTION

1976 Census question.

15. Is the person handicapped by a *serious* long-term illness or physical or mental condition? • If yes, tick the appropriate boxes for each person to show types of handicap. • If not handicapped tick box 8. • If no illnesses or conditions tick box 8.	In his or her education.........................	☐1
	In getting or holding a job..................	☐2
	In getting about alone.........................	☐3
	In doing housework............................	☐4
	In sporting or recreational activities..	☐5
	In acts of daily living, e.g. dressing, bathing................................	☐6
	In other ways.....................................	☐7
	Not handicapped................................	☐8

APPENDIX 2. – SURVEY OF DISABILITY, AGEING AND CARERS 1998 DISABILITY CRITERIA

Disability

A person has a disability if he/she has one of the following that has lasted or is likely to last for 6 months or more:

- loss of sight (not corrected by glasses);
- loss of hearing (with difficulty communicating or use of aids);
- loss of speech;
- chronic or recurring pain that restricts everyday activities;
- breathing difficulties that restrict everyday activities;
- blackouts, fits or loss of consciousness;
- difficulty learning or understanding;
- incomplete use of arms or fingers;
- difficulty gripping;
- incomplete use of feet or legs;
- a nervous or emotional condition that restricts everyday activities;
- restriction in physical activities or physical work;
- disfigurement or deformity;
- needing help or supervision because of a mental illness or condition;
- head injury, stroke or other brain damage, with long-term effects that restrict everyday activities;
- treatment for any other long-term condition, and still restricted in everyday activities or
- any other long-term condition that restricts everyday activities. □

Specific restrictions are:

- core activity restrictions and/or
- schooling or employment restrictions.

Core activities are:

- self care – bathing or showering, dressing, eating, using the toilet and managing incontinence;
- mobility – moving around at home and away from home, getting into or out of a bed or chair and using public transport;
- communication – understanding and being understood by others: strangers, family and friends.

Core activity restriction may be:

- profound – unable to perform a core activity or always needing assistance;
- severe – sometimes needing assistance to perform a core activity;
- moderate – not needing assistance, but having difficulty performing a core activity and
- mild – having no difficulty performing a core activity, but using aids or equipment because of disability.

APPENDIX 3

September 1998 test : form type 4: yes/no response.

For developing health policies and community based programs, it is important to measure the extent of disability existing in Australia.

18. Mark YES or NO for each of the following: Does the person have difficulty ...		
• doing everyday activities such as eating, showering or dressing?	☐ Yes	☐ No
• hearing?	☐ Yes	☐ No
• learning, understanding or remembering things?	☐ Yes	☐ No
• reading or seeing even with glasses?	☐ Yes	☐ No
• walking, kneeling or climbing stairs?	☐ Yes	☐ No
• living independently?	☐ Yes	☐ No
• doing any other things people of the same age usually do (for example working, studying, etc.)	☐ Yes	☐ No

19. What causes the difficulty shown in Q18 for the person?

☐ Short-term health condition (lasting less than 6 months)
☐ Long-term health condition
☐ Disability
☐ Age
☐ Difficulty with English language
☐ Other cause – please specify
☐ ☐ ☐ ☐ ☐ ☐ ☐ ☐ ☐
☐ ☐ ☐ ☐ ☐ ☐ ☐ ☐ ☐
☐ ☐ ☐ ☐ ☐ ☐ ☐ ☐ ☐
☐ No difficulty

APPENDIX 4

September 1998 test: form type 5: scaled response.

For developing health policies and community-based programs, it is important to measure the extent of disability existing in Australia.

18. How much difficulty does the person have in:	None	A little	A lot
• doing everyday activities such as eating, showering or dressing?	☐	☐	☐
• hearing?	☐	☐	☐
• learning, understanding or remembering things?	☐	☐	☐
• reading or seeing even with glasses?	☐	☐	☐
• walking, kneeling or climbing stairs?	☐	☐	☐
• living independently?	☐	☐	☐
• doing any other things people of the same age usually do (for example working, studying, etc.)	☐	☐	☐

19. What causes the difficulty shown in Q18 for the person?

☐ Short-term health condition (lasting less than 6 months)
☐ Long-term health condition
☐ Disability
☐ Age
☐ Difficulty with English language
☐ Other cause – please specify
☐☐☐☐☐☐☐☐
☐☐☐☐☐☐☐☐
☐☐☐☐☐☐☐☐
☐ No difficulty

APPENDIX 5

Table A5.1. Census Test September 1998: Form Type 4 – Percentage of Selected Demographic Characteristics by Selected Census Population Groups.

	Matched Disability (%)	False Positive (%)	False Negative (%)	Matched Non-Disability (%)	All Persons (%)	Total No.
Form type 4						
Age						
0–14 years	3.6	2.1	2.8	91.5	100.0	471
15–59 years	6.1	3.3	8.2	82.4	100.0	1,672
60 years and over	25.5	9.7	17.4	47.4	100.0	683
All persons	10.4	4.6	9.5	75.5	100.0	2,826
Sex						
Males	10.6	5.0	8.6	75.8	100.0	1,343
Females	10.1	4.3	10.4	75.2	100.0	1,483
All persons	10.4	4.6	9.5	75.5	100.0	2,826
Birthplace						
Australian, NZ, UK, North America, South Africa	9.3	3.7	8.1	79.0	100.0	2,301
Other European	17.2	9.8	16.7	56.3	100.0	419
Northeast, Southeast and Southern Asian	7.1	4.8	2.4	85.7	100.0	42
Middle East and North Africa	9.1	0.0	0.0	90.9	100.0	11
Other countries	5.0	15.0	15.0	65.0	100.0	20
Not answered	9.1	3.0	24.2	63.6	100.0	33
All persons	10.4	4.6	9.5	75.5	100.0	2,826
All persons (no.)	293	131	269	2,133	2,826	2,826

Table A5.2. Census Test September 1998: Form Type 5 – Percentage of Census Population Groups by Selected Demographic Characteristics.

	Matched Disability (%)	False Positive (%)	False Negative (%)	Matched Non-Disability (%)	All Persons (%)	Total No.
Form Type 5						
Age						
0–14 years	3.6	5.2	5.6	21.0	16.1	461
15–59 years	28.2	39.8	50.2	65.1	56.7	1,626
60 years and over	68.1	55.0	44.1	14.0	27.3	782
All persons	100.0	100.0	100.0	100.0	100.0	2,869
Sex						
Males	50.6	51.9	45.1	47.6	48.2	1,382
Females	49.4	48.1	54.9	52.4	51.8	1,487
All persons	100.0	100.0	100.0	100.0	100.0	2,869
Birthplace						
Australian, NZ, UK, North America, South Africa	70.6	79.2	73.7	85.2	81.8	2,346
Other European	25.5	17.3	21.6	10.8	14.2	408
Northeast, Southeast and Southern Asian	1.2	2.2	1.4	1.5	1.5	43
Middle East and North Africa	0.2	0.0	0.0	0.2	0.2	5
Other countries	0.7	0.4	1.4	0.6	0.7	19
Not answered	1.7	0.9	1.9	1.7	1.7	48
All persons	100.0	100.0	100.0	100.0	100.0	2,869
All persons (no.)	411	231	213	2,014	2,869	2,869

Table A5.3. Census Test September 1998: Form Type 5 – Percentage of Selected Demographic Characteristics by Selected Census Population Groups.

	Matched Disability (%)	False Positive (%)	False Negative (%)	Matched Non-disability (%)	All Persons (%)	Total No.
Form type 5						
Age						
0–14 years	3.3	2.6	2.6	91.5	100.0	461
15–59 years	7.1	5.7	6.6	80.6	100.0	1,626
60 years and over	35.8	16.2	12.0	35.9	100.0	782
All persons	14.3	8.1	7.4	70.2	100.0	2,869
Sex						
Males	15.1	8.7	6.9	69.3	100.0	1,382
Females	13.7	7.5	7.9	71.0	100.0	1,487
All persons	14.3	8.1	7.4	70.2	100.0	2,869
Birthplace						
Australian, NZ, UK, North America, South Africa	12.4	7.8	6.7	73.1	100.0	2,346
Other European	25.7	9.8	11.3	53.2	100.0	408
Northeast, Southeast and Southern Asian	11.6	11.6	7.0	69.8	100.0	43
Middle East and North Africa	20.0	0.0	0.0	80.0	100.0	5
Other countries	15.8	5.3	15.8	63.2	100.0	19
Not answered	14.6	4.2	8.3	72.9	100.0	48
All persons	14.3	8.1	7.4	70.2	100.0	2,869
All persons (no.)	411	231	213	2,014	2,869	2,869

APPENDIX 6

Example of a possible 'need for assistance' census disability question.

For developing health policies and community based programs, it is important to measure the extent of disability existing in Australia.

18. Does the person ever need someone to help with, or be with them, for any of the following activities:	Yes, always	Yes, sometimes	No
• doing everyday activities such as eating, showering, dressing or toileting?[a]	☐	☐	☐
• getting out of bed, moving around at home or going to or getting around places away from home?[a]	☐	☐	☐
• understanding or being understood by others?[a]	☐	☐	☐
• household chores such as laundry, vacuuming or dusting?	☐	☐	☐
• meal preparation?	☐	☐	☐
• home maintenance or gardening tasks?	☐	☐	☐

19. What is the reason for the need for assistance or supervision shown in Q18 for the person?

- ☐ Short-term health condition (lasting less than 6 months)
- ☐ Long-term health condition (lasting 6 months or more)
- ☐ Disability
- ☐ Effects of ageing
- ☐ Child too young
- ☐ Difficulty with English language
- ☐ Other cause – please specify

  ....

  ....
- ☐ No difficulty

[a]Activities which comprise ABS 'core activity restriction'.

APPENDIX 7

Proposed 'Core activity support needs' questions for Australian 2006 National Census of Population and Housing.

26. Does the person ever need someone to help with, or be with them for self-care activities? For example, doing everyday activities such as eating, showering, dressing or toileting.	() Yes, always () Yes, sometimes () No
27. Does the person ever need someone to help with, or be with them for body movement activities? For example, getting out of bed, moving around at home or at places away from home.	() Yes, always () Yes, sometimes () No
28. Does the person ever need someone to help with, or be with them for, communication activities? For example, understanding, or being understood by, others.	() Yes, always () Yes, sometimes () No
29. What are the reasons for the need for any assistance or supervision shown in questions 26, 27 and 28? Mark all applicable reasons.	() Short-term health condition (lasting less than 6 months) () Long-term health condition (lasting 6 or months or more) () Disability (lasting 6 months or more) () Old or young age () Difficulty with English language () Other cause () No need for help or supervision

Questions 26, 27 and 28 identify 'core' activities where assistance is needed. Question 29 identifies the reason(s) for any need for assistance identified in the previous questions and acts as a filter for output purposes. Note that only a 'yes, always' or 'yes, sometimes' response to any of Questions 26, 27 or 28 when combined with a reason in Question 29 of 'Long-term health condition', 'Disability' or 'Old or young age and age greater than 40 years' will place a person in the 'core activity support needs' output category.

Reasons of 'short-term health condition', 'young age', difficulty with English language' or 'other' will by themselves exclude the person from the 'core activity need for assistance' output population.

Appendix 7 was not included in the original paper, but has been added as a postcript to inform readers of more recent developments.

PARTICIPATION AND ENVIRONMENT: OUT OF THE MELTING POT AND INTO ...?

Ros Madden

1. INTRODUCTION

The International Classification of Functioning, Disability and Health (ICF) was published in 2001 after over a decade of international discussion and field testing (see, for instance, Bickenbach, Chatterji, Badley, & Ustun, 1999). Its ratification by the World Health Assembly was keenly awaited in Australia, by people interested in working with a model of disability attuned to a human rights and equal opportunities approach, and by people wanting to use the new model in disability and health policy and information systems. This paper outlines developments being implemented and ideas being discussed in Australia, particularly with the Australian Collaborating Centre (ACC).[1]

The paper contains a brief outline of the ICF, and then focuses on the Participation and Environment components of the ICF. In order to implement these ICF components, it is necessary to think about:

- the single list of domains of Activities and Participation and options for using them,
- qualifiers, or measures, which are recognised as being essential to meaningful application, and
- the Environment component, and how to record it.

International Views on Disability Measures: Moving Toward Comparative Measurement
Research in Social Science and Disability, Volume 4, 225–246

ISSN: 1479-3547/doi:10.1016/S1479-3547(05)04012-1

The ICF is intended to be a multi-purpose classification and the paper includes a brief discussion of applications, including the adoption of ICF into Australian data standards. In focusing on measurement – the theme of the session – there is an underlying emphasis on the use of the ICF in information systems capable of producing meaningful data on disability.

2. OVERVIEW OF THE INTERNATIONAL CLASSIFICATION OF FUNCTIONING, DISABILITY AND HEALTH

The ICF defines functioning and disability as multi-dimensional concepts, relating to:

- the body functions and structures of people
- the Activities people do and the life areas in which they Participate
- the factors in their Environment that affect these experiences.

Each of these components is defined in the context of a health condition. Disability is the umbrella term for any or all of: an impairment of body structure or function, a limitation in Activities or a restriction in Participation.

In the ICF, a person's functioning or disability is conceived as a dynamic interaction between health conditions and environmental and Personal Factors (see Figure 1). Environmental Factors – an important new component of the ICF – are included in recognition of their influence on functioning and disability. Although Personal Factors are recognised in the interactive model shown in Figure 1, they are not classified in, and are beyond the scope of, the ICF. Such factors might include age, sex and indigenous status and would be selected by users according to the application.

2.1. Definitions

The following are definitions of the components:

- *Body functions* are the physiological functions of body systems (including psychological functions).
- *Body structures* are anatomical parts of the body such as organs, limbs and their components.
- *Impairments* are problems in body function and structure such as significant deviation or loss.

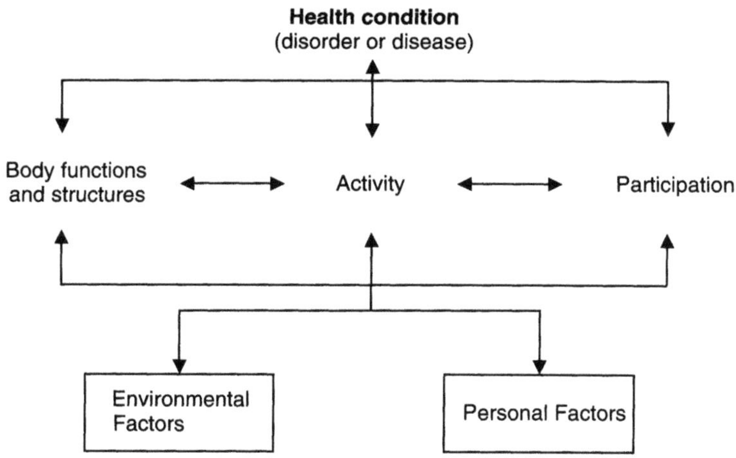

Fig 1. Interactions Between Components of the ICF. *Source:* WHO 2001:18.

- *Activity* is the execution of a task or action by an individual.
- *Participation* is involvement in a life situation.
- *Activity limitations* are difficulties an individual may have in executing Activities.
- *Participation restrictions* are problems an individual may experience in involvement in life situations.
- *Environmental Factors* make up the physical, social and attitudinal environment in which people live and conduct their lives. These are either barriers to or facilitators of the person's functioning.

2.2. Domains, Classifications and Codes

Each component is composed of various domains; these are sets of related physiological functions, anatomical structures, actions, tasks, areas of life and external influences. The ICF has a separate chapter for each of the domains. Table 1 lists ICF components and domains, with examples of some of the contents of each domain. The ICF contains a hierarchy of classifications and codes for each of the components – Body Functions and Structures, Activities and Participation and Environmental Factors. In information systems, these codes may be recorded (using up to four digits) to indicate the body, Activity or Participation domains affected.

Table 1. ICF Components and Domains, with Examples of Contents.

Component	Domains (Chapter Headings) with Examples of Contents
Body functions: eight chapters	Mental functions, e.g. memory function, intellectual functions
	Sensory functions and pain, e.g. hearing function, smell function
	Voice and speech functions, e.g. articulation functions
	Functions of the cardiovascular, haematological, immunological and respiratory systems, e.g. blood pressure functions, respiratory muscle functions
	Functions of the digestive, metabolic and endocrine systems, e.g. ingestion functions, endocrine gland functions
	Genitourinary and reproductive functions, e.g. menstruation functions
	Neuromusculoskeletal and movement-related functions e.g mobility of joint functions
	Functions of the skin and related structures, e.g. repair functions of the skin
Body structures: eight chapters	Structures of the nervous system, e.g. spinal cord and related structures
	The eye, ear and related structures, e.g. structure of eyeball and inner ear
	Structures involved in voice and speech, e.g. structure of mouth
	Structures of the cardiovascular, immunological and respiratory systems
	Structures related to the digestive, metabolic and endocrine systems, e.g. structure of intestine gall bladder and ducts
	Structures related to the genitourinary and reproductive systems, e.g. structure of the urinary system and pelvic floor
	Structures related to movement, e.g. structure of head and neck region
	Skin and related structures, e.g. structure of skin glands
Activities & participation: nine chapters	Learning and applying knowledge, e.g. learning to read, solving problems
	General tasks and demands, e.g. carrying out daily routine
	Communication, e.g. speaking, conversation
	Mobility, e.g. getting around inside or outside home
	Self-care, e.g. washing oneself, dressing
	Domestic life, e.g. preparing meals, acquiring a place to live
	Interpersonal interactions and relationships, e.g. relating with strangers, formal relationships, family relationships
	Major life areas, e.g. work and employment, remunerative employment
	Community, social and civic life, e.g. recreation and leisure, religion and spirituality
Environmental factors: five chapters	Products and technology, e.g. products and technology for communication; design, construction and building products and technology of buildings for public use
	Natural environment and man-made changes to environment, e.g. physical geography, light, sound, air quality
	Support and relationships, e.g. immediate family, health professionals
	Attitudes, e.g. individual attitude of friends and health professionals
	Services, systems and policies, e.g. social security services, systems and policies

2.3. Qualifiers

Measures can be recorded against each of the neutral codes, to indicate the extent of 'problem' with any of these aspects of functioning. Environmental Factors can be recorded as being either barriers to, or facilitators of, a person's functioning.

These 'qualifiers' are numeric measures coded after the relevant category code. Qualifiers are recognised as essential to the meaningful use of the classification because the domains and codes are expressed in neutral language. Without qualifiers, the codes have no inherent meaning (WHO, 2001, p. 222).

A uniform or 'generic' qualifier is provided to record the extent of the 'problem' in relation to impairment, Activity limitation, Participation restriction and environmental barrier. The extent of the problem is denoted using the following scale:

Generic qualifier:

0	No problem
1	Mild problem
2	Moderate problem
3	Severe problem
4	Complete problem
8	Not specified
9	Not applicable

The Environmental Factor qualifier uses both a positive and a negative scale to indicate the extent to which an Environmental Factor acts as either a facilitator or barrier.

Qualifier for Environmental Factors:

.0	No barrier	+0	No facilitator
.1	Mild barrier	+1	Mild facilitator
.2	Moderate barrier	+2	Moderate facilitator
.3	Severe barrier	+3	Substantial facilitator
.4	Complete barrier	+4	Complete facilitator
.8	Barrier, not specified	+8	Facilitator, not specified
.9	Not applicable	+9	Not applicable

2.4. Performance and Capacity

Two constructs – 'performance' and 'capacity' – can also be used with the generic qualifiers for the Activities and Participation domains. These constructs essentially categorise the environment, in which measurement is taking place, into two classes. According to the ICF (WHO, 2001, p. 15):

> *performance*...describes what an individual does in his or her current environment;
>
> *capacity*...describes an individual's ability to execute a task or an action...(and) aims to indicate the highest probable level of functioning that a person may reach in a given domain at a given moment. To assess the full ability of the individual, one needs a 'standardised' environment to neutralise the varying impact of different environments on the ability of the individual. This 'standardised' environment may be (a) an actual environment commonly used for capacity assessment in test settings; or (b) in cases where this is not possible, an assumed environment which can be thought to have a uniform impact.

The ICF also states:

> The gap between capacity and performance reflects the difference between the impacts of current and uniform environments, and thus provides a useful guide as to what can be done to the environment of the individual to improve performance (WHO, 2001, p. 15).

Thus, the notion of 'capacity' also relates to the identification of what is needed to enhance a person's opportunities to 'perform' to their 'highest probable level of functioning'. In this sense, the 'assumed' environment may be thought of as, in some sense, optimum. This aspect of the concept of 'capacity' appears to accord with Australian policy goals, focusing on people's abilities. In comparison, the notion of a 'standardised environment' may be more difficult to operationalise widely, and there is no experience to illustrate how this can reliably be done.[2]

Much of this debate about operationalising capacity is yet to be resolved.

The ICF is intended to be grounded in a human rights philosophy, and its relationship to the *UN standard rules on equalization of opportunities for persons with disabilities* is acknowledged. Operationalising these rules appears to relate primarily to performance, i.e. the *actual* Participation experience of people with disabilities.

The existence of these two constructs emphasises, perhaps imperfectly, the environmental component of the ICF model: it is impossible to record a person's disability without describing and measuring the environment. If environment is adequately recorded, it may then not be important to name one performance in one environment as 'capacity' and another, in another environment, as the actual 'performance'.

Rather, it can be seen that there is a large spectrum of possible functional performance for any individual, highly dependent on the environment at the time.

3. ACTIVITIES, PARTICIPATION AND ENVIRONMENT: MEASUREMENT

How, then, do we begin to use the ICF to 'measure' Activities and Participation?

3.1. Activities and Participation: Using the Single List

The classification provides a single list of Activity and Participation domains, or life areas, with options for use. WHO reflects several years of difficulty in reaching consensus on a definitive separation of two lists of Activities and Participation domains, when it states that (WHO, 2001, p. 16):

> It is difficult to distinguish between Activities and Participation on the basis of domains.... Therefore ICF provides a single list that can be used if users wish to do so to differentiate Activities (A) and Participation (P) in their own operational ways.... Basically there are four possible ways of doing so:
>
> (a) to designate some domains as A and others as P, not allowing any overlap,
> (b) same as (a) above, but with partial overlap,
> (c) to designate all detailed domains as A and use the broad category headings as P, and
> (d) to use all domains as both A and P.

Activities and Participation are, then, two separate concepts in the ICF, with distinct definitions, but measured along the same domains.

3.2. Draft Criteria for Delineating Activities and Participation

The delineation of the concepts of Activity and Participation has been a consistent goal of the ACC and its advisers. Criteria for distinguishing the two concepts, in line with their definitions in the final ICF, were accordingly developed, revised and discussed during the process of ICF development and testing.

The ACC draft criteria for distinguishing Activities and Participation are included in the Australian User Guide for use and comment:

i. Activities focus on the person's individual functioning, while Participation emphasises the person's involvement in society.

ii. A is completely externally observable. P refers to the 'lived experience of the person' (WHO, 2001, p. 15).
iii. Activity *can* relate to a 'test' environment (although it can also relate to a 'real' environment), with or without equipment. Participation is essentially 'confounded' with the environment, i.e. the concept has little meaning without consideration of the physical and social environment, and it cannot be 'assessed' in a 'test' environment. 'Involvement in society' relates in particular to societal roles. This highlights the confounding of Participation with that part of the environment that shapes expected roles and societal norms.
iv. A is fine-grained whereas P is broad-brushed.
v. A is about action or process, P relates to the overall goal of actions or sets of actions.

These draft criteria expand on the WHO definitions (see Section 2). Both definitions and draft criteria could be applied, together, in delineating Activities and Participation in practice. The purpose is either to

- split the A–P domains, so that some apply to Activities and the others to Participation, i.e. option (a) and
- use the A–P domains with partial or total overlap, together with qualifiers, in order to achieve delineated approaches to Activities and Participation, i.e. option (b) or (d).

The ACC attempted to find a split of the A–P domains that it could endorse, for general adoption of option (a) in Australia, but this proved not possible (see AIHW, 2003a, pp. 36–38; see also CIHI, 2001). We concluded that

- The ACC is not able at this stage to recommend a split of the domains for general use; that is, it is not able to recommend option (a) as a general solution to delineating Activities and Participation.
- Option (a) may nevertheless be suitable for specific applications, where users can obtain agreement among stakeholders on a suitable split of the domains, consistent with the ICF definitions. Users are invited to record their experience in the template in Australian User Guide (AIHW, 2003a).

3.3. Using the Qualifiers as the Basis for Delineating Activities and Participation – Options (b) and (d)

If potential users preserve separate concepts of Activities and Participation, does it matter if they wish to use and interpret the domains somewhat differently in different circumstances? Is it in fact more useful to use the freedom offered in options (b) and (d) to adapt and experiment in this difficult area?

It is logically obvious that if any domain can be used for *either* Activities or Participation, then the delineation between Activities and Participation must involve the use of different qualifiers, as the only other tools available in the classification for this purpose.

In ICF terms, this means that if options (b) or (d) are adopted, then the 'generic qualifier' must be translated into suitable language for Activities and Participation separately, and/or additional qualifiers must be provided, such as a qualifier for Participation, indicating 'involvement in life situations' (see 'additional qualifiers' above, in Section 2). In Australia we have therefore worked to provide qualifiers that

- can be used to help delineate Activities from Participation for ICF users using option (b) or (d),
- can also be used with option (a), and
- are consistent with the ICF.

3.4. Qualifiers for Activities

The ICF gives us:

- Activities domains.
- A qualifier about 'difficulty' with the Activity (the generic qualifier); the statement is made that difficulty can be measured with or without assistive devices or personal assistance, and as capacity or performance; the constructs of performance and capacity relate to the person in a specified environment.
- Environmental Factors that may facilitate or be a barrier to the Activity.

Further, a great deal of service planning and provision relies in practice on the notion of 'need'. Need relates to Environmental Factors (such as personal assistance, equipment, environmental modifications) that may be present in the standardised or 'optimum' environment but are not in the current environment (where current performance is achieved). What has emerged from discussion in our Advisory Committee on Australian and International Disability Data (ACAIDD) is the need to operationalise more explicitly a concept of 'Assistance with Activity'. This is considered to be an important subset of Environmental Factors on which much measurement work has been done, and a major component of disability and aged care services policy in Australia.[3] Work to date conceptualises 'Assistance with Activity' as a multidimensional concept, relating to the duration, frequency and intensity of assistance; information on various scales in use is being assembled. This qualifying concept would be used to describe aspects of the (current, or standardised, or optimum) environment, in terms commonly used in measurement and assessment tools – i.e. to record more detail than just 'with or without assistance' as currently envisaged in the ICF. Thus, this concept would be consistent with the ICF and would supplement the information obtained by using the ICF. It is planned to continue work on this idea.

Two possible qualifiers for Activities are therefore suggested: the ICF generic qualifier ('difficulty') and a second qualifier based on the qualifying concept suggested above ('Assistance with Activity'). These measures can be used in different environments; each could, of course, result in different measures, depending on which environment is present.

3.5. Qualifiers for Participation

Work has been carried out in Australia on the measurement of Participation, both during the revision years and since publication of the ICF in May 2001. Two qualifiers have been developed – 'Participation extent' and 'Participation – satisfaction level'. A review of measures of Participation confirmed these ideas as appropriate templates for the development of data elements for the National Community Services Data Dictionary V3 (AIHW, 2003b; see also Bricknell & Madden, 2002).

The qualifier 'Participation extent' corresponds to the ICF generic qualifier and indicates the extent of Participation restriction. This corresponds to an externally observable (or 'objective') measure of Participation.

The qualifier 'Participation – satisfaction level' corresponds to the person's own perspective on their Participation, and reflects their attitude to their Participation in the various life domains. It is essentially a summary measure in which the concepts of satisfaction, choice, opportunity and importance are embedded. This corresponds to the qualifier for 'involvement or subjective satisfaction' allowed for in the ICF (WHO, 2001, p. 231, Annex 2). Such a qualifier may indicate a 'performance gap' for Participation, in that a person may indicate life areas where they are not satisfied, and may indicate Environmental Factors that could ameliorate the situation.

3.6. The E Dimension and its Qualifiers

How do the ideas, outlined so far, fit with the Environmental Factors? Because of the definitions of Activity and Participation, information about them (including the qualifiers) is not meaningful without the Environmental Factors also being coded. This is, of course, in line with the ICF model and the philosophy that disability is largely environmentally determined. The rising reported prevalence of attention deficit hyperactivity disorder (ADHD) illustrates this point. Can we adequately report on such changes in prevalence without also being able to quantify changes in school organisation, community tolerance of certain behaviours, as well as changes in medical practices, pharmaceutical resources and the rates of prescribing of related drugs?

WHO offers three coding conventions for Environmental Factors, namely to code factors:

(a) as they affect the person overall,
(b) as they broadly affect each of Body Structure and Function, Activity and Participation, and
(c) against every single Body Function, Body Structure, Activity and Participation code used.

Beta testing in Australia generally revealed reluctance for the third option, not only because it was very labour intensive, but also because of the duplication involved – a number of Environmental Factors occurred repeatedly as impacting on more than one code in another dimension. Nevertheless there may be applications where it will be important to relate each Environmental Factor to each individual impairment, Activity limitation or Participation restriction. There may be other applications where one of the other two options may provide information adequate to the purpose.

The qualifiers of the Environmental Factors are well conceptualised. Because of their newness, it will be important systematically to record and share information and experience as they come into more and more common use. As practice builds up, calibration will be important here too.

The more general challenge is to ensure that we use this new aspect of the classification to its fullest extent and, each time we use the classification, to ask whether we have adequately incorporated Environmental Factors into our applications.

4. THE 'INFORMATION MATRIX'

WHO states that the information gathered from the list of Activities and Participation, suitably qualified, provides an information matrix, recording performance and capacity in each of the life domains (WHO, 2001, p. 14). If option (b) or (d) is adopted, then an expanded information matrix is created.

If, for instance, users opted to use the qualifiers described above, to delineate Activities and Participation, then codes for both Activities and Participation would be recorded in the following format: [4]

- *axxxx*.$q_p q_c$—the first qualifier being difficulty with Activity in the current environment and the second being difficulty in a standard or optimum environment; if qualifiers for assistance are developed, these would be additional.
- *pxxxx*.$q_p q_c$—the first qualifier would relate to extent of Participation and the second to Participation in an optimum (or standard) environment; if qualifiers for satisfaction are developed, these would be additional.

Table 2. Expanded Information Matrix for Option (b) – Some of A–P Overlap.

	Qualifiers							
	Performance				Capacity			
	Activity		Participation		Activity		Participation	
Domains	Difficulty	Assistance	Extent	Satisfaction	Difficulty	Assistance	Extent	Satisfaction
Learning and applying knowledge								
General tasks and demands								
Communication								
Mobility								
Self-care								
Domestic life								
Interpersonal interactions and relationships								
Major life areas								
Community, social and civic life								

Key: (shading is illustrative only, not a recommended split of the domains)

	Domains less likely to relate to Participation
	Domains that may relate to Activities or Participation
	Domains less likely to relate to Activities

As outlined above, these qualifiers (recorded measures) can only be interpreted if the environment is also recorded – whether the environment is current, optimum or standard, and whether it is a facilitator or barrier (using the qualifiers offered by the ICF).

The expanded matrix could then look like Table 2 (drawn to correspond to option (b)).

5. IMPLEMENTATION IN AUSTRALIA: NATIONAL DATA STANDARDS AND DISABILITY SERVICES

The ICF is a multi-purpose classification designed to serve many sectors and disciplines across different countries and cultures.

Our work in Australia on ICF development was shaped early on by people attending a 1994 Australian workshop on the ICIDH and the measurement of disability. They identified a wide range of people and purposes that would benefit from national consistency in disability concepts and measurement (AIHW, 1994)

- consumers interested in ways of better relating data on needs for services and the provision of services,
- service providers and planners interested in relating needs, eligibility criteria and resource allocation,
- people and policy makers interested in equity and wanting agreed broad definitions of disability in order to define and monitor exclusion and inclusion,
- clinicians of many disciplines who wished to relate disability outcomes and the 'severity' of functioning to appropriate interventions, and to relate their clinical practice to experience in the wider population,
- national and international statisticians interested in being able to estimate prevalence (the proportion of the population with a disability), needs for support and outcomes in informative and comparable ways (it was noted that the ICIDH had already been widely used to develop national surveys in Australia and elsewhere),
- policy makers in a wide range of fields (e.g. aged care, insurance, compensation and income security) who wished to improve their data and to be able to relate it to data collected in other fields.

This section first outlines how such national consistency is being supported in Australia, and then discusses a specific application.

5.1. National Data Standards

The AIHW is Australia's national agency for health and welfare statistics and information, as well as the ACC for the WHO Family of International Classifications. We work on national data development, collection, analysis, dissemination and publication. In the area of national data development we work with and support nationally constituted data committees, under national information agreements that oblige all Australian jurisdictions, the Institute and the ABS to work to develop and exchange national data on health, housing and community services.

Two of the main products resulting from these efforts are the national data dictionaries for health and for community services (e.g. AIHW, 2003b, c). These are major pieces of national information infrastructure. They contain national information models, and associated data elements, specified in accord with ISO standards. The dictionaries provide a menu of data items from which national minimum data sets (MDSs) can be specified, relating to the major national collections in these fields.

The Institute's involvement in the ICF development stemmed from all aspects of our national role, but most obviously our responsibilities for national data development. The ICF offers us the chance to increase the consistency of disability data within Australia, which is a high priority.

Data elements have been developed to operationalise the ICF concepts in Australian data collections, including qualifiers that enable us to adopt options (b) and (d) for Australian use of Activities and Participation. These data elements have been published in AIHW (2003b) and will appear in the new on-line metadata registry (METeOR) in mid-2005.

5.2. A National Data Set on Disability Support Services

A practical application of the ICF has been implemented in a national MDS for disability support services in Australia. The Institute worked with senior disability administrators in the nine Australian jurisdictions to develop a national data set for disability support services provided under the Commonwealth State/Territory Disability Agreement (CSTDA). This is a national programme (with total funding of approximately $3 billion in 2002–2003) for people with ongoing support needs, over 50% of whom have an intellectual disability as their primary disability. It was considered that there are two main areas of the CSTDA MDS where the ICF can usefully be applied: 'A + P support needs' and Participation outcomes.

5.2.1. Activity and Participation (A+P) Support Needs

Because the disability support services provided under the CSTDA may address any area of Activities and Participation, and because any area of A and P may affect the intensity of support needed, there appears to be no need to split the single list for the 'support needs' question in the CSTDA MDS. What is required, rather, is to:

- Group the A and P chapters so that the groupings are meaningful and not too onerous for service delivery agencies to fill in. Retain the combined 'A and P' name, as it does not seem necessary (in an information sense) to say whether the support provided is directed to A or P, but rather to the life area (A + P domain) where support is provided.
- Qualify the domains – this will be done using the concepts of difficulty and assistance in a way that maintains consistency with the ABS population survey (e.g. ABS, 1999); these are interpreted as performance related.

Table 3 depicts the information to be sought on support needs.

5.2.2. Participation Outcomes

A 'Participation module' was developed as a long-term outcome measure (see Table 4). The over-arching goal of the CSTDA is to improve the quality of life for people with disabilities by improving their Participation. Accordingly, the Participation domains chosen for this purpose must reflect the broad human rights focus of the CSTDA. At this stage it is envisaged that:

- Service funders and providers can use this Participation module for purposes, such as client review at various stages, overall assessments of quality of life, overall service and needs planning, periodic client satisfaction surveys. The module would produce data as comparable and as possible to those collected in the broader population survey (e.g. ABS, 1999). The 'qualifiers' concord with those in the National Community Services Data Dictionary (AIHW, 2003b), based on quite extensive research and development (e.g. Bricknell and Madden, 2002; AIHW, 2003a, d).
- The module will provide a high-level framework into which more service-specific outcomes (related to service specific goals) can be mapped. This will ensure that the service specific outcome indicators relate to the overall CSTDA outcome indicators and thence to some population measures.[5]

Table 3. Support Needs Question from the CSTDA NMDS.

11. How often does the service user need personal **help** or **supervision** with **activities** or **participation** in the following life areas? *See Data Guide page 62*

Please indicate the level of help or supervision required for each life area (rows a–i) by ticking only one level of help or supervision (columns 1–5).

The person can undertake activities or participate in this life area with this level of personal help or supervision (or would require this level of help or supervision if the person currently helping were not available) **LIFE AREA**	1) Unable to do or always needs help/ supervision in this life area	2) Sometimes needs help/ supervision in this life area	3) Does not need help/ supervision in this life area but uses aids or equipment	4) Does not need help/ supervision in this life area and does not use aids or equipment	5) Not applicable
a) Self-care e.g. washing oneself, dressing, eating, toileting	☐ 1	☐ 2	☐ 3	☐ 4	
b) Mobility e.g. moving around the home and/or moving around away from home (including using public transport or driving a motor vehicle), getting in or out of bed or a chair	☐ 1	☐ 2	☐ 3	☐ 4	
c) Communication e.g. making self understood, in own native language or preferred method of communication if applicable, and understanding others	☐ 1	☐ 2	☐ 3	☐ 4	
d) Interpersonal interactions and relationships e.g. actions and behaviours that an individual does to make and keep friends and relationships, behaving within accepted limits, coping with feelings and emotions	☐ 1	☐ 2	☐ 3	☐ 4	
NOTE: *In the following questions '**not applicable**' is a valid response **only if** the person is 0–4 years old.*					
e) Learning, applying knowledge and general tasks and demands e.g. understanding new ideas, remembering, problem solving, decision making, paying attention, undertaking single or multiple tasks, carrying out daily routine	☐ 1	☐ 2	☐ 3	☐ 4	☐ 5
f) Education e.g. the actions, behaviours and tasks an individual performs at school, college, or any educational setting	☐ 1	☐ 2	☐ 3	☐ 4	☐ 5
g) Community (civic) and economic life e.g. recreation and leisure, religion and spirituality, human rights, political life and citizenship, economic life such as handling money	☐ 1	☐ 2	☐ 3	☐ 4	☐ 5
NOTE: *In the following questions '**not applicable**' is a valid response **only if** the person is 0–14 years old.*					
h) Domestic life e.g. organising meals, cleaning, disposing of garbage, housekeeping, shopping, cooking, home maintenance	☐ 1	☐ 2	☐ 3	☐ 4	☐ 5
i) Working e.g. actions, behaviours and tasks to obtain and retain paid employment	☐ 1	☐ 2	☐ 3	☐ 4	☐ 5

Source: AIHW 2004, AIHW 2003a.

Table 4. Draft 'Participation Outcomes framework'.

Life area	Extent of participation (judged by service provider or assessment process)	Satisfaction with participation (judged by consumer, with advocate if necessary) in relation to duration, frequency, manner or outcome
	1. Full participation 2. Mild participation restriction 3. Moderate participation restriction 4. Severe participation restriction 5. Complete participation restriction	1. High satisfaction with participation 2. Moderate satisfaction with participation 3. Moderate dissatisfaction with participation 4. Extreme dissatisfaction with participation 5. No participation 6. No participation and none desired
Participation in communication and conversation (e.g. producing and receiving spoken, nonverbal, formal sign or written messages, involvement in conversation, discussion with or without use of communication devices and techniques)		
Participation in mobility within the home and community environment (e.g. changing and maintaining body position; carrying, moving and handling objects; walking and moving; moving around using transportation)		
Participation in domestic life (e.g. acquiring necessities such as a place to live and goods and services; household tasks such as preparing meals; caring for household objects and assisting others)		
Participation in interpersonal interactions and relationships (e.g. relating with strangers, formal and informal social relationships, family and intimate relationships)		
Participation in education, work and employment (e.g. informal education, preschool, school, vocational and higher education; work preparation such as apprenticeships; acquiring, keeping and terminating a job, remunerative or non-remunerative employment)		
Participation in economic life (e.g. basic and complex economic transactions, economic self-sufficiency)		
Participation in community, social and civic life (e.g. community life, religion and spirituality, recreation and leisure, political life and citizenship, human rights)		

Source: AIHW 2004, AIHW 2003a.

6. DISCUSSION AND CONCLUSION: INTERNATIONAL CLASSIFICATION OF FUNCTIONING, DISABILITY AND HEALTH IMPLEMENTATION CHALLENGES

The ICF has significant implications for national and international data collections, both in terms of the content and scope of the collections. Successful implementation in information systems requires decisions on the use of the Activities and Participation domains, on their qualifiers, and on a determined introduction of Environmental Factors into many human service information systems that do not currently record such information.

6.1. Overview

This paper has focussed on 'measurement' and the recording of Activity and Participation outcomes and Environmental Factors. Three main points have been made.

- To operationalise the separate concepts of Activities and Participation, separate measures or 'qualifiers' should be used for each; a general solution to splitting the single list of domains to delineate Activities and Participation does not appear achievable.
- The separate qualifiers are allowed for in the ICF and are now reflected in Australian data standards and in use in data systems. If the ICF is to fulfil its promise, to facilitate the collection of more relevant and more consistent data on disability, then translating ICF into national data standards, as described in Section 5, may also be a useful example of implementation.
- Environmental Factors must be recorded. These are a fundamental part of the ICF model, critical to understanding Activities and Participation. If Environmental Factors are adequately recorded, there is no need to wrestle with operationalising the construct of 'capacity'.

6.2. Discussion: The Importance of Recording and Sharing Experience

The Activities and Participation qualifiers are located in the broad and busy field of measurement and assessment. Many existing assessment tools are in use, and are embedded in measurement and even payment methods in services around Australia (and around the world). In Australia, some basic mapping has been undertaken in the disability data development described above, to confirm the feasibility of collecting data as Table 3. Much more of this kind of work is needed.

There are a range of measurement issues that need consideration in any ICF measurement application (Madden, 1999), including:

- the need to clarify purpose before deciding method,
- the importance of understanding the role played by 'perception' in measurement (i.e. who measures – sometimes oversimplified as a distinction between 'objective' and 'subjective'), and
- the vital role played by people with disabilities in the ICF revision and the hope that this more inclusive model of development would permeate the other members of the WHO 'family of classifications'.

These three issues remain important during ICF implementation.

The new ICF is likely to prove invaluable as a conceptual and information-oriented framework for a wide range of applications relating to human functioning. These applications may be about to expand significantly. It will be important to build up knowledge about measurement, and its purpose, method and the impact of the perspective of the measurer. Progress is important because of the persisting possibility that some applications, particularly those with large resources, will swamp those that move more slowly or are less adequately resourced.

Annex 3 of the ICF concludes with a statement recognising that practice must be built up, recorded and analysed regarding the 'operationalisation' of Activities and Participation. The ICF is a valuable resource, it needs more work to be put into practice, and implementation experience needs to be shared.

In order to harness and harmonise the rapid progress that is now likely to occur, a development schema would appear to be useful.[6] The goal of such a schema would be to promote coherent ongoing development, and consistency where that is achievable, and it could include something like:

- criteria, principles and protocols for the use of the Activity and Participation dimensions, depending on which of the WHO options is chosen by the user,
- a template for recording experience, purpose, practice and reasoning so as to facilitate the exchange of information about development in all four areas discussed in this paper,

- guidelines for calibration, refining, mapping and relating of existing measures and assessment tools to the ICF, and for the development of new ones,
- methods of sharing and publishing results, to promote discussion, quality and consistency.

Internationally with the development of the ICF, we undertook and finished an exhaustive and exciting process. Collectively we developed, tested and argued shared ideas, and tried to seek common ground in the interests of a more valuable and inspirational classification. We now have a new classification. It seems likely that we must continue our collaborative work and our vigorous discussions.

In this spirit, I look forward to receiving comments on this paper.

NOTES

1. This paper has been revised and updated since 2001, reflecting developments since then; in particular it reflects material now published in the ICF Australian User Guide (AIHW, 2003a), which used and refined the ideas of the 2001 version of this paper. Members of the Advisory Committee on Australian and International Disability Data contributed to the development of the User Guide. A number of people in the ACC provided stimulating comments on this paper and/or the User Guide, including Richard Madden, Ching Choi, Catherine Sykes, Louise York, Samantha Bricknell, Paul Magnus, Trish Ryan and Diane Gibson. The paper contains the views of the author and does not necessarily represent those of the ACC.

2. The 'construct' of 'capacity in a standardised environment' appears to relate to a conceptualisation of health that distinguishes between 'within the skin' factors and external factors. This distinction in turn relies on the notion of a separate individual with intrinsic capacity, where better health outcomes can be promoted by health interventions and environmental modifications. This approach is said to reflect an egalitarian, human rights philosophy. In practice it provides extreme challenges to measurement. Conceptually, it also appears at odds with the more organic or ecological inter-relationships pictured in the ICF diagram.

The need to introduce the idea of 'capacity' into the classification is driven at least in part by the desire to measure the effectiveness of health systems and how well they are closing the gap between capacity and performance. This purpose brings with it the need to define and confine the scope of the health system, not holding it accountable for measures that, while promoting good human health and functioning, are beyond the scope of many health systems. This aim of assessing health systems, thus may lead to the search for a measurement of 'capacity'. But looking at effectiveness of these systems also requires the measurement of human outcomes – that is, the level of health and human functioning (to indicate the 'performance gap'). We are then faced again with the need to attribute some of this gap to the health system, illustrating that perhaps the use of the 'capacity' construct has not solved the problem for which it was introduced.

3. The presence of information on 'assistance' in many assessment and measurement tools was reported by Van Buuren, Hopman-Rock, and Miedema (1996). 'Assistance' is also a key concept in the Australian disability survey (see e.g ABS, 1999).

4. The 'xxxx' in the example indicates that up to four digits may be used to record the precise area of Activity or Participation being affected.

5. For instance, one of the CSTDA high-level goals could be interpreted to be increasing participation in employment. Participation outcomes for CSTDA clients could be compared to the rest of the population by ensuring that the high-level participation module uses national data items, such as labour force status (used in labour force surveys and in the ABS disability survey). Service-specific goals for employment services are articulated as helping people get jobs, and the existing indicators agreed between service funders and providers record the number of jobs gained over a period, the duration of jobs, etc.

6. The AIHW (in its User Guide on its website) now provides some opportunity for information sharing among users and feedback in its role as ACC; WHO is, in 2005, piloting a format for information exchange and feedback on its website.

REFERENCES

Australian Bureau of Statistics (ABS). (1999). *Disability, ageing and carers: Summary of findings* Cat. no. 4430.0. Canberra: ABS.

(Australian Institute of Health and Welfare). AIHW. (1994). *Measurement of disability: Workshop proceedings* Canberra, Australia, 21–22 February 1994. Canberra: AGPS.

Australian Institute of Health and Welfare (AIHW). (2003a). ICF Australian user guide. Version 1.0. Disability series. AIHW Cat No. DIS 33. Canberra: AIHW (see also http://www.aihw.gov.au).

Australian Institute of Health and Welfare (AIHW). (2003b). *National community services data dictionary.* Vesrion 3. Canberra: AIHW.

Australian Institute of Health and Welfare (AIHW). (2003c). *National health data dictionary* Vesrion 3. Canberra: AIHW.

Australian Institute of Health and Welfare (AIHW). (2003d). *Australia's national disability services data collection: Redeveloping the commonwealth-state/territory disability agreement national minimum data set* AIHW cat. no. DIS 30. Canberra: AIHW.

Australian Institute of Health and Welfare. (2004). *Data guide: Data items and definitions* 2003–04 (CSTDA NMDS). Canberra: AIHW.

Bickenbach, JE., Chatterji, S., Badley, EM., & Ustun, TB. (1999). Models of disablement, universalism and the international classification of impairments, disabilities and handicaps. *Social Science Medicine*, *48*, 1173–1187.

Bricknell, S., & Madden, R. (2002). Exploring the measurement of participation. Paper presented at WHO-FIC meeting, Brisbane, 14–20 October 2002.

Canadian Institute for Health Information (CIHI) (2001). Development of mutually exclusive lists for activities and participation: WHO international classification of functioning, disability and health. Viewed September 2002, http://www.secure.cihi.ca/cihiweb/en/downloads/codingclass_icidh_e_FinalDraftAP.pdf.

Madden, R. (1999). May the ICIDH be with you – the potential force of the ICIDH in Australia. Paper for the 6th annual meeting of the NACC for ICIDH, Vancouver, October 1999.

Van Buuren S., Hopman-Rock M., & Miedema H. S. (1996). *The development of a proposal for revision of the severity of disabilities scale of the ICIDH.* TNO report PG 96.067, Leiden, The Netherlands.

World Health Organization. (2001). *International classification of functioning, disability and health (ICF).* Geneva: WHO.

THE IMPACT OF ASSISTIVE DEVICE USE ON DISABILITY MEASUREMENT

Elizabeth K. Rasch, Barbara M. Altman and Jennifer H. Madans

ABSTRACT

National estimates of persons with disability are of great importance since they inform policy and program development. However, accurate estimation depends on accurate measurement, and disability measurement is still evolving. Using data from the 1994–1995 National Health Interview Survey and Disability Supplement, this study examines the relationship between functional and activity limitations and equipment use in order to characterize the influence of environmental factors on disability measurement. Our findings highlight the challenging methodologic issues related to measuring a concept of disability that reflects person–environment interactions.

INTRODUCTION

Estimates of the population of persons with disability, and characteristics of this population, are critical to the development of health and social policy.

International Views on Disability Measures: Moving Toward Comparative Measurement
Research in Social Science and Disability, Volume 4, 247–262

ISSN: 1479-3547/doi:10.1016/S1479-3547(05)04013-3

At the national level, this information is used to inform public policy in the areas of resource allocation, service provision, prevention, and equalization of opportunities. However, identifying disability through empirical measurement requires a conceptualization of disability and operational definitions linking those concepts to measurements (Altman, 2001). At the conceptual level, disability has been recognized as a process rather than a state, defined as the product of the interaction between persons with potentially disabling conditions and their environment (Brandt & Pope, 1997).

Translating such a concept into measures suitable for large-scale surveys poses a methodological challenge. How can biological, environmental, and socially constructed components of the disablement process, as well as their interaction, be captured empirically? Altman notes that most conceptual models of disability do not suggest methods of operationalization for empirical measurement (Altman, 2001). While the International Classification of Impairments, Disabilities, and Handicaps (ICIDH), now called the International Classification of Functioning and Disability (ICF, World Health Organization, 2001), offers a detailed schema to code information related to disability, its usefulness is dependent on the development of measurement tools that are congruous with the conceptualization of disability framing the classification (Altman, 2001). According to Altman, the missing element in linking concepts of disability to empirical measurement is an operational definition of disability that tells us what to observe and how to describe it (Altman, 2001).

What elements should comprise an operational definition of disability? Representing the Quebec Committee on the ICIDH, Fougeyrollas proposes consideration of the characteristics of a person's impairments (specification of what body structures and functions are impaired) and disabilities (as represented by functional limitations, such as mobility or learning problems) resulting from disease, trauma, or congenital causes, and environmental characteristics comprised of social and ecological factors (Fougeyrollas, 1995). In the proposed taxonomy of environmental factors, technology is included as an ecologic element. Self-reported use of assistive technology (AT) is one environmental feature that has been collected in national health surveys, allowing exploration of its effect on disability measurement. Use of AT has been shown to reduce the need for personal assistance (Allen, Foster, & Berg, 2001; Hammel, Lai, & Heller, 2002), and to reduce or eliminate difficulty performing tasks (Verbrugge, Rennert, & Madans, 1997). However, it is not known how AT use interacts with other definitional elements such as indicators of impairment, functional, or activity limitation, or how it effects disability estimation from national surveys.

Using data from the 1994–1995 National Health Interview Survey (NHIS) and its associated Disability Supplement, this study examines the relationship between functional and activity limitations and equipment use in order to begin to characterize the influence of environmental factors on disability measurement. Specifically, we wish to know the proportion of persons with functional limitations who report use of assistive devices and, more importantly, whether persons who are successfully adapting to their functional limitations through use of AT are reporting those underlying limitations.

METHODS

Data source: The NHIS is a continuous nationwide survey of the U.S. civilian non-institutionalized population by household interview using a multistage probability sampling design. In 1994–1995, the survey included a disability supplement (NHIS-D) to address the shared need of Federal agencies for national information on disability. The NHIS-D was conducted in two phases, performed at different times, to reduce respondent burden. Phase I was administered at the same time as the NHIS core survey, and collected basic data on disability on all members of the NHIS households. Phase II was conducted after Phase I and collected additional information about specific subpopulations or additional detail on specific aspects of disability. Responses to questions on the NHIS core and NHIS-D, Phase I were used for this analysis. Over-sampling of African-Americans (1994, 1995) and Hispanic persons (1995) was performed to improve the precision of prevalence estimates for these subgroups. Detailed descriptions of the NHIS and NHIS-D survey design, sampling method, and plan of operation have been reported elsewhere (Adams & Marano, 1995; Benson & Marano, 1998).

Subjects: The interviewed sample for 1994 and 1995 included 107,469 and 95,091 persons, respectively, for a total sample of 202,560. The overall response rate for the NHIS core and Phase I of the Disability Supplement was 87%. For the purpose of this paper, the analysis was limited to adults, age 18 years and older, yielding a total analytic sample of 145,007 persons.

Variables of interest: Demographic data included sex, age, education, annual family income, employment status, marital status, and health status. Respondent age (18–44, 45–64, >65 years), annual family income (<$20,000, $20,000–49,999, >$50,000), education (<high school, high school, >high school), employment status (employed, not employed, not in labor force), and health status (excellent/very good, good, fair/poor) were categorized as indicated for analysis. Marital status was recoded for analysis as married, widowed, divorced/separated, or never married. Responses of "married, spouse in household" and "married, spouse not in household" were included as married.

The presence of functional limitation was determined by responses to questions about difficulty lifting 10 pounds, climbing 10 stairs, walking a quarter of a mile, standing for 20 minutes, bending to pick up an object on the floor, reaching, holding a pen or pencil, and grasping (Table 1). Respondents were classified as having a functional limitation (dichotomous variable) if they reported inability or difficulty performing one or more of the eight functional actions. Respondents were classified as having a lower extremity functional limitation if they reported inability or difficulty with one or more of the five (of eight) functional actions that primarily required use of the lower extremities (lifting, stair climbing, walking, standing, or bending). All remaining respondents were classified as not having a functional limitation or lower extremity functional limitation. Less than 1% of the responses to each one of the eight functional limitation variables were missing ("refused," "don't know," and "not ascertained" responses). Using the method described above, it was possible to classify the functional limitation status of all respondents, including those with missing responses to some variables.

Self-reported limitations in activities of daily living (ADL), instrumental activities of daily living (IADL), or major activities (i.e. work) were used to characterize activity limitations. For ADLs and IADLs, respondents were asked about the need for help, special equipment, a reminder, and the degree of difficulty accomplishing these tasks (Table 1). ADL tasks included bathing/showering, dressing, eating, getting in or out of a bed or chair, using the toilet, and walking inside the home. IADL tasks included meal preparation, shopping, managing money, using the phone, and performing light housework. Although respondents were asked about their ability to perform heavy housework, these responses were not included in the analysis of IADL limitations. In a factor analysis, Fleishman, Spector, and Altman (Fleishman, Spector, & Altman, 2002) found that heavy housework reflected a factor distinct from the other IADL categories and was commonly the only task limitation mentioned by a large component of the sample. Respondents were classified as having an ADL or IADL limitation (dichotomous variables) if they reported inability, difficulty, or the need for help or supervision performing one or more of the six ADL tasks or one or more of the five IADL tasks, respectively.

Table 1. Examples of Questions from the NHIS-D Survey Used to Classify Functional Limitations, Activity Limitations, Equipment Use, and Disability Identity.

Category	Example Questions
Functional limitations	"Do you have any difficulty lifting something as heavy as 10 pounds, such as a full bag of groceries?" "How much difficulty do you have lifting 10 pounds, some, a lot, or are you completely unable to do this?"
Activity limitations	
ADL	"Because of a physical, mental, or emotional problem, do you get help from another person in dressing?" "Because of a physical, mental, or emotional problem, do you need to be reminded to dress or need to have someone close by when you do it?" "Do you have difficulty dressing?" "How much difficulty do you have dressing, some, a lot, or are you unable to do it?"
IADL	"Because of a physical, mental, or emotional problem, do you get help or supervision from another person with preparing your own meals?" "Do you have any difficulty preparing your own meals?" "How much difficulty do you have preparing your own meals, some, a lot, or are you unable to do it?"
Major activity	"What were you doing most of the past 12 months; working at a job, keeping house, going to school, or something else?" "Does any impairment or health problem now keep you from working (doing housework, etc.)?" "Are you limited in the kind or amount of work (housework, etc.) you can do because of any impairment or health problem?" "Are you limited in any way in any activities because of an impairment or health problem?"
Non-sensory equipment use	"Do you now use any of these aids to get around (a cane, crutches, walker, medically prescribed shoes, a wheelchair, a scooter)?" Which aids do you use? "Have you used or are you expected to use (aid identified) for 12 months or longer?"
Disability identity	"Do you consider yourself to have a disability?" "Would other people consider you to have a disability?"

To identify limitations in major life activities, respondents were asked a series of questions about limitations in work, keeping house, school, or other activities (Table 1). The specific questions that respondents received were based on their age and self-reported usual activity. For the purposes of this study, respondents were categorized with a major activity limitation (dichotomous variable) if they indicated inability or limitation performing their major activity or limitation in another activity.

A dichotomous variable reflecting the presence or absence of activity limitation was created using the recoded (dichotomous) indicators of ADL, IADL, and major activity limitation described above. Persons with one or more limitations in major activities, ADL, or IADL variables were classified as having an activity limitation.

Non-sensory equipment use was determined from responses to questions about use of mobility devices, braces, prostheses, and ADL equipment (Table 1). These questions were asked independently of questions on functional and activity limitation status such that all adults were queried about non-sensory equipment use regardless of whether they reported limitations. Mobility device use was identified by affirmative responses to questions about use of a cane, crutches, walker, medically prescribed shoes, a wheelchair, or a scooter. Similarly, brace users were identified by affirmative responses to these questions: "Does anyone in the family now use a brace of any kind? Who is this? On what part of the body is the brace worn? Is it worn on the back, neck, arm, hand, leg, foot, or knee?" In addition, respondents were asked about use of prostheses (artificial leg, foot, arm, or hand) and ADL equipment (special equipment used for bathing, dressing, eating, getting in/out of bed or chairs, toileting, and getting around inside the home).Self-reported duration of equipment use was available for mobility aids and braces. This information was used to classify respondents as temporary (expect to use device <12 months) versus long-term (expect to use device ≥ 12 months) equipment users. Use of prostheses and ADL equipment was assumed to be long-term.

Questions about use of special listening devices (telephone amplifier, telecommunications device for the deaf/ teletypewriter (TDD/TTY) or teletype, closed caption TV, etc.) and special visual equipment (telescopic lenses, braille, readers, etc.) were only asked of persons reporting trouble hearing or seeing for more than 12 months. Since questions about sensory AT use were only asked of persons with self-reported sensory limitations (with the exception of hearing aid use), it could not be determined if there were sensory AT users who did not report sensory limitations, and therefore, use of sensory AT could not be included in these analyses.

An indicator of disability identity designated respondents who considered themselves to have a disability (self-identity) or who thought other people considered them to have a disability (other-identity) (Table 1). Proxy responses were classified as missing for the analysis of disability identity.

Data Analysis

Prevalence estimates and standard errors (SE) were determined for limitations in functional tasks, ADL, IADL, and major activities, as well as equipment use. Functional limitations were cross-classified with equipment use to determine the proportions of persons who used AT but did not report functional limitations. In addition, functional limitations were cross-classified with AT use in persons with and without activity limitations (presence or absence of ADL, IADL, or major activity limitation). From this analysis, two proportions were calculated: (1) the proportion of persons using AT on a long-term basis who reported functional limitations but did not report activity limitations and (2) the proportion of persons using AT on a long-term basis who did not report either functional or activity limitations. Prevalence estimates and SE values for socio-demographic variables were calculated for the total adult population, for persons who reported functional or activity limitations and were long-term AT users, and for persons who did not report limitations but used AT on a long-term basis. Estimates were based on a minimum of 30 responses per analytic cell with relative SE values less than 30%. Sample weights were used to produce population estimates by adjusting for differential selection probability from sampling methods (over-sampling), non-coverage, and non-response. Variance estimation was accomplished via Taylor linearization using software designed to take into account the complex sampling design (SUDAAN).

RESULTS

The prevalence (and SE) of functional limitations and lower body functional limitations among adults 18 years of age and older was 13.2% (0.14) and 12.2% (0.13), respectively. Of the eight types of functional limitation, difficulty or inability walking a quarter of a mile was reported most frequently (7.7% + 0.10). Activity limitation was identified by one or more self-reported ADL, IADL or major activity limitations. The prevalence (SE) of activity limitations among adults was 18.5% (0.16) overall; the percent reporting ADL, IADL, and major activity limitations were 2.5% (0.05), 3.7% (0.06), and 18.1% (0.16), respectively. The prevalence of any limitation, which combines non-sensory functional limitation and activity limitation indicators to identify persons who report any form of limitation, was 21.7% (0.18).

The prevalence of temporary and long-term non-sensory equipment use by adults 18 years of age and older in the U.S., according to type of device, is shown in Table 2. Long-term non-sensory device use was more prevalent 4.7% (0.07) than temporary device use 1.0% (0.03). Among non-sensory AT users, mobility device use was reported most frequently. In adults with activity limitations (those who reported ADL, IADL, or major activity limitations), the prevalence of long-term and temporary non-sensory device use was 20.7% (0.27) and 3.1% (0.12), respectively.

Relationships between functional limitations and AT use are shown in Table 3. In Panel A, mobility device use among those with and without lower body functional limitations is described. Of those who used mobility devices on a long-term basis, 13.1% (0.52) did not report lower body functional limitations. Most of these individuals reported use of canes or medically prescribed shoes. However, some manual wheelchair users as well as other mobility device users reported no lower body functional limitations. In Panel B, the relationship between brace use and functional limitations is described. Of those who used braces on a long-term basis, 37.0% (1.14) did not report any functional limitation. Most of these individuals reported use of back or knee braces. Of those who used prostheses or ADL equipment,

Table 2. Prevalence (% (SE)) of Assistive Technology Use among Adults.

	Long-Term AT Users	Temporary AT Users
Mobility devices[a]	3.1 (0.05)	0.8 (0.03)
ADL equipment	1.3 (0.04)	*
Braces[b]	1.5 (0.04)	0.6 (0.02)
Prostheses[c]	0.1 (0.01)	*
Any non-sensory equipment[d]	4.7 (0.07)	1.0 (0.03)

Note: *Indicates duration of use not asked of respondents.
[a]Includes canes, crutches, walkers, medically prescribed shoes, wheelchairs, and scooters.
[b]Includes back, neck, arm, hand, leg, foot, knee, or other brace use.
[c]Includes artificial legs, feet, arms, or hands.
[d]Combines mobility, brace, prosthetic, and ADL equipment indicators to identify persons who report use of any type of non-sensory equipment.

Table 3. Relationships between Functional/Activity Limitation and Use of Assistive Technology.

		Percent (SE)[a] not reporting lower body functional limitation[b]	Percent (SE) reporting lower body functional limitation
Panel A	Mobility device use[c]		
	Not a device user	90.7 (0.11)	9.3 (0.11)
	Long-term device user	13.1 (0.52)	86.9 (0.52)
	Temporary device user	23.9 (1.31)	76.1 (1.31)
		Percent (SE) not reporting functional limitation[d]	Percent (SE) reporting functional limitation
Panel B	Brace use[e]		
	Not a brace user	87.8 (0.13)	12.2 (0.13)
	Long-term brace user	37.0 (1.14)	63.0 (1.14)
	Temporary brace user	53.0 (1.86)	47.0 (1.86)
		Percent (SE) not reporting functional limitation	Percent (SE) reporting functional limitation
Panel C	Prosthetic use[f]		
	Not a prosthetic user	86.9 (0.14)	13.1 (0.14)
	Prosthetic user	30.1 (4.02)	69.9 (4.02)
		Percent (SE) not reporting ADL limitation[g]	Percent (SE) reporting ADL limitation
Panel D	ADL equipment use		
	Not a device user	98.5 (0.04)	1.5 (0.04)
	Device user	19.6 (1.01)	80.4 (1.01)

[a]SE = standard error.
[b]Lower body functional limitations include self-reported inability or difficulty lifting, climbing stairs, walking a quarter of a mile, standing for 20 minutes, or bending.
[c]Includes canes, crutches, walkers, medically prescribed shoes, wheelchairs, and scooters.
[d]Functional limitations include self-reported inability or difficulty lifting, climbing stairs, walking a quarter of a mile, standing for 20 minutes, bending, reaching, holding a pen or pencil, and grasping.
[e]Includes back, neck, arm, hand, leg, foot, knee, or other brace.
[f]Includes artificial legs, feet, arms, or hands.
[g]ADL limitations include self-reported inability, difficulty, or the need for help or supervision with bathing/showering, dressing, eating, getting in or out of a bed or chair, using the toilet, or walking inside the home.

Table 4. Percent Distribution of Assistive Technology Use and Percent Distribution of Functional Limitation Status by Assistive Technology Use Stratified by Activity Limitation Status (Presence or Absence of ADL, IADL, or Major Activity Limitations).

		(% SE)		
		No AT use	Long-term AT use	Temporary AT use
No activity limitations	**Total (100%)**	**98.5 (0.04)**	**1.0 (0.04)**	**0.5 (0.02)**
	No functional limitation	96.5 (0.1)	65.2 (1.3)	73.6 (1.9)
	Functional limitation	3.5 (0.1)	34.8 (1.3)	26.4 (1.9)
		100%	100%	100%
Activity limitations	**Total (100%)**	**76.2 (0.3)**	**20.7 (0.3)**	**3.1 (0.1)**
	No functional limitation	56.3 (0.4)	11.8 (0.5)	22.0 (1.5)
	Functional limitation	43.7 (0.4)	88.2 (0.5)	78.0 (1.5)
		100%	100%	100%

Table 5. Percent (SE) of Adults who were Long-Term AT Users without Reported Functional or Activity Limitations by Type of Non-Sensory Assistive Technology (AT) Used.

Self-Reported Type of AT Use[a]	Proportion of Adults Using AT Long-Term without Functional or Activity Limitations
Knee braces	23.4 (1.8)
Back braces	21.2 (1.6)
Canes	18.6 (1.5)
Other long-term equipment[b]	13.3 (1.3)
Medically prescribed shoes	13.3 (1.3)
Leg and foot braces	7.0 (1.2)
Hand braces	4.2 (0.8)
Arm braces	4.2 (0.8)

[a]Proportions do not add to 100% because respondents may have reported use of more than one type of equipment.
[b]Other long-term equipment includes self-reported long-term use (12 months or more) of crutches, walkers, manual and electric wheelchairs, scooters, ADL equipment, neck braces, prostheses, and other braces.

30.1% (4.02) and 19.6% (1.01) respectively, did not report associated functional (Panel C) or ADL limitations (Panel D).

Functional limitations were cross-classified with AT use in persons with and without activity limitations (Table 4). Among those with no activity limitation (no ADL, IADL, or major activity limitations), 1% used AT on a long-term basis and of those, 34.8% (1.34) reported functional limitations but, more importantly, 65.2% (1.34) did not report functional limitations. The majority of these persons used braces, canes, or medically prescribed shoes (Table 5). For instance, 23.4% (1.8) of long-term AT users who did not report functional or activity limitations used knee braces; 21.7% (1.73) used knee braces exclusively (i.e. no other equipment use was reported). Similarly, 21.2 (1.6) of long-term AT users without reported functional or activity limitations used back braces and 19.1% (1.62) used back braces exclusively. However, there were manual wheelchair users and other long-term device users who reported no functional or activity limitations (Table 5). If the proportion of persons who did not report activity limitations (ADL, IADL, or major activity limitations) but used non-sensory AT on a long-term basis are added to the population of persons with activity limitations, they comprise 4.2% of the new population.

Socio-demographic characteristics of persons who reported no functional or activity limitations but who used AT on a long-term basis are described in Table 6. The group was predominantly male, 18–44 years old, had greater than a high school education and a family income over $20,000, were married, employed, and reported very good or excellent health status. Of this group, only 3.9% (0.71) of self-respondents considered themselves to have a disability and only 3.7% (0.75) thought others would consider them to have a disability. This contrasts with persons reporting functional or activity limitations who are long-term AT users, as 43.4% (0.75) of this group considered themselves to have a disability and 39.7% (0.74) thought others would consider them to have a disability.

DISCUSSION

In this study, the proportions of civilian, non-institutionalized adults in the U.S. who do not report activity limitations, but who used AT on a long-term basis were identified. Delineation of this subgroup highlights the dynamic and interactional nature of disability, a process in which adaptation to long-term health events can affect function. This poses a challenge for disability measurement. In the biological sense, adaptation can be thought of as alteration in

Table 6. Sociodemographic Characteristics of Long-Term AT Users (Adults).

	Distribution% (SE)[a]		
	Total population of adults	AT users reporting functional or activity limitations	AT users not reporting functional or activity limitations
Age			
18–44	56.8	18.7	51.0
45–64	26.8	26.1	23.0
65+	16.4	55.2	26.0
Gender			
Male	47.8	42.0	55.3
Female	52.2	58.0	44.7
Education[b]			
<12 years	19.1 (0.21)	38.4 (0.70)	17.1 (1.53)
High school	37.2 (0.21)	33.7 (0.67)	36.7 (1.95)
>High school	43.8 (0.30)	28.0 (0.67)	46.1 (2.11)
Family income[b]			
<\$20,000	27.4 (0.31)	54.1 (0.88)	32.1 (1.92)
\$20,000–49,999	44.6 (0.30)	34.5 (0.77)	42.5 (2.37)
\$50,000+	28.0 (0.34)	11.4 (0.56)	25.3 (2.15)
Employment status			
Employed	65.1 (0.22)	17.1 (0.61)	65.2 (1.96)
Unemployed	2.9 (0.06)	1.6 (0.17)	2.5 (0.67)
Not in labor force	32.0 (0.22)	81.3 (0.63)	32.4 (1.96)
Marital status[b]			
Married	64.1 (0.23)	47.4 (0.74)	61.0 (1.86)
Widowed	6.9 (0.08)	29.3 (0.65)	12.0 (1.30)
Divorced/separated	9.8 (0.10)	13.0 (0.39)	10.8 (1.27)
Never married	19.2 (0.22)	10.2 (0.49)	16.2 (1.45)
Health status[b]			
Excellent/very good	62.0 (0.25)	16.1 (0.54)	59.9 (1.92)
Good	25.4 (0.19)	26.1 (0.61)	30.2 (1.79)
Fair/poor	12.7 (0.14)	57.9 (0.75)	9.9 (1.09)

[a]SE values are not reported for age and gender because these data are post-stratified to the U.S. Census.

[b]Missing values excluded (<1.4% for education, <16.9% for family income, <0.2% for marital status, and <0.9% for health status).

the structure or function of an organism to become better suited to survive in its environment (Stein, 1980). Alternatively, it can be thought of as the process by which a person maintains a useful relationship to the environment when conditions for accomplishing everyday activities have changed (Thoren-Jonsson, Moller, & Grimby, 1999; Thoren-Jonsson, 2001; White, 1974). This process involves the alignment of personal goals and abilities with physical, social, and environmental demands on the individual (Thoren-Jonsson et al., 1999). Since individuals and environments are constantly changing, adaptive processes are dynamic. In the presence of health conditions and/or impairments, use of AT represents one form of adaptation employed to optimize safety, autonomy, and functioning. Reduction in personal assistance and improved ability to perform tasks have been attributed to AT use (Allen et al., 2001; Hammel et al., 2002; Verbrugge et al., 1997).

What does this mean for disability measurement? If persons accommodate to impairments (such as through the use of AT) thereby eliminating limitations, should they be counted among those with a disability? This paper identified a relatively small proportion of persons who did not report ADL, IADL, or major activity limitations but used non-sensory AT on a long-term basis. When added to the population of persons with ADL, IADL, or major activity limitations, these persons comprised 4.2% of the population of persons with "disabilities." Since this subpopulation did not report activity limitations, they were identified by self-reported use of non-sensory AT. Of the numerous ways in which persons may adapt to impairments, it is likely that use of non-sensory AT represents the tip of an iceberg. Using qualitative research methods, Thoren-Jonsson described 18 strategies used by persons with physical impairments resulting from poliomyelitis to accomplish every day activities (Thoren-Jonsson et al., 1999). Examples of adaptive strategies include stretching the limits of physical capacity, developing new techniques to accomplish tasks, prioritizing daily activities, restoring role balance by engaging in new or different activities, orchestrating daily tasks by coordinating with others, and compensation through use of objects in the environment. National estimates of the number of persons with disability are affected if adaptive strategies such as these result in prevention or elimination of functional and activity limitations. If public health interventions and anti-discrimination laws, programs, or policies were to maximize accommodations and opportunities for persons with disability, such as through implementation of the Americans with Disabilities Act, the relatively small proportion of persons we identified in this analysis through their use of AT, that were not identified by activity limitation measures, would be much larger. The impact of how this might change the identification of those with disabilities depends on how disability is defined and the intended use of the data.

Thus, in order to be fully informative, an interactional definition of disability calls for a more complex approach to this subpopulation. This subpopulation includes persons with impairments who are experiencing limitations whether or not they use assistive devices, have a supportive environment, or have plentiful resources. It also includes persons with impairments who may not experience limitations because they have made adaptations to enable their participation. The latter group could be considered at higher risk than the general population for restrictions in activities and/or participation since they may experience limitations in unsupportive environments (i.e. those without necessary accommodations). In order to determine the effectiveness of services, accommodations, or equalization of opportunities intended to enhance the participation of persons who report limitations, the elaboration of the population must include those who have the potential for experiencing limitations but have successfully accommodated, in addition to those currently experiencing restrictions in participation. Services, programs, policies, and laws would be deemed effective if the proportion of persons who are participating fully in everyday life due to successful accommodations increased while the proportion of persons experiencing limitations decreased. Thus, the response to the request for the identification of the disabled population requires two parts: (1) the fit between individual characteristics and the environment taking into account all current accommodations and (2) the fit without accommodations (or where accommodations have not been developed). It is important to identify which population is relevant for the specific question at hand. As accommodations become more available and successful, the difference between these two populations will increase.

In this analysis, persons who used non-sensory AT on a long-term basis without reported functional or activity limitations were predominantly male, young, employed, married, with above average education, income, and health status. In many respects, they resembled the general adult population with the exception of self-reported long-term use of AT. It is important to note that some of these respondents used wheelchairs, walkers, scooters, and prostheses. However, the majority reported use of braces, canes, or medically prescribed shoes. Thus, it can be argued that adults who reported use of back and knee braces for instance, but did not report limitations are probably active, healthy adults who only use these devices for leisure, sport, or work activities. However, the data indicate that the majority of persons who reported exclusive use of back or knee braces (without reported limitations) were not employed in occupations that would require the use of such braces for injury prevention (such as construction or freight handling). This suggests that brace use may have been the result of some previous injury or impairment. Should this group be counted among those with a disability? Current conceptual models acknowledge disability as a process that occurs along a continuum, influenced by factors within and outside of the individual (Brandt & Pope, 1997; Nagi, 1991). Yet, national efforts to estimate the number of persons with disabilities seek to classify this human variation into a simple dichotomy. If disability occurs along a continuum, then it should be recognized that different estimates (using different cut-points or definitions) are needed to serve different programmatic or policy-driven purposes and that no single estimate of the disabled population will address all purposes. Thus, determination of whether or not to include persons reporting use of back or knee braces, but not limitations, in disability estimates would be based on the purpose of measurement.

Strengths of this study include a large analytic sample that was nationally representative of the civilian, non-institutionalized adult population. Questions about non-sensory AT use, and limitations in activities and function were asked of all adults. Thus, information on non-sensory AT use was obtained not only from those who reported a limitation, but also from those who did not report limitations. However, our analysis had to be limited to the subpopulation of persons using non-sensory AT since, in the 1994–1995 NHIS-D, questions about sensory AT use were only asked of persons with self-reported sensory limitations (with the exception of hearing aid use). Therefore, it could not be determined if there were sensory AT users who did not report functional limitations. Thus, it is important for survey instruments to separate descriptors of functioning and the environmental milieu so that potential interactions can be determined. An additional limitation of the study is the small number of measures reflecting the environment. Since AT represents one of many possible accommodations that persons with impairments might utilize to optimize their participation, the population of persons with disability is probably underestimated in national surveys if the purpose is to identify the number of persons who may benefit from accommodations and equalization of opportunities.

In summary, this analysis identified the proportion of civilian, non-institutionalized adults in the U.S. who did not report activity limitations, but who used AT on a long-term basis. A person–environment interactional definition of disability would suggest that adaptive processes such as AT use and/or other environmental factors might have positively influenced the participation of these individuals. This raises questions about the purposes of disability measurement, how to operationalize interactional definitions of disability, how to deal with adaptation to long-term health events at the empirical level, and the practicality of implementing adequate measures of the environment in national surveys.

REFERENCES

Adams, P. F., & Marano, M. A. (1995). Current estimates from the National Health Interview Survey, 1994. *Vital Health Statistics*, *10*(193), 1–3, 130–141. National Center for Health Statistics.

Allen, S. M., Foster, A., & Berg, K. (2001). Receiving help at home: The interplay of human and technological assistance. *The Journals of Gerontology. Series B, Psychological Sciences and Social Sciences*, *56*(6), S374–S382.

Altman, B. A. (2001). Disability definitions, models, classification schemes, and applications. In: G. L. Albrecht, K. D. Seelman & M. Bury (Eds), *Handbook of disability studies* (pp. 97–122). Thousand Oaks, CA: Sage Publications.

Benson, V., & Marano, M. A. (1998). Current estimates from the National Health Interview Survey, 1995. *Vital Health Statistics*, *10*(199), 1–3, 125–136. National Center for Health Statistics.

Brandt, E. N. Jr., & Pope, A. M. (1997). Models of disability and rehabilitation. In: N. B. Edward, Jr. & M. P. Andrew (Eds), *Enabling America (assessing the role of rehabilitation science and engineering)* (pp. 62–80). Washington, DC: Institute of Medicine, National Academy Press.

Fleishman, J. A., Spector, W. D., & Altman, B. M. (2002). The impact of differential item functioning on age and gender differences in functional disability. *Journal of Gerontology, Social Sciences*, *57B*(5), 275–284.

Fougeyrollas, P. (1995). Documenting environmental factors for preventing the handicap creation process: Quebec contributions relating to ICIDH and social participation of people with functional differences. *Disability and Rehabilitation*, *17*(3–4), 145–153.

Hammel, J., Lai, J.-S., & Heller, T. (2002). The impact of assistive technology and environmental interventions on function and living situation status with people who are ageing with developmental disabilities. *Disability and Rehabilitation*, *24*(1–3), 93–105.

Nagi, S. Z. (1991). Disability concepts revisited: Implications for prevention. In: M. P Andrew & R. T. Alvin (Eds), *Disability in America* (pp. 309–327). Washington, DC: Institute of Medicine, National Academy Press.

Stein, J. (Ed.). (1980). The random house college dictionary (Revised edition) (p. 15). New York: Random House, Incorporated.

Thoren-Jonsson, A. L. (2001). Coming to terms with the shift in one's capabilities: A study of the adaptive process in persons with poliomyelitis sequelae. *Disability and Rehabilitation*, *23*(8), 341–351.

Thoren-Jonsson, A. L., Moller, A., & Grimby, G. (1999). Managing occupations in everyday life to achieve adaptation. *The American Journal of Occupational Therapy*, *53*(4), 353–362.

Verbrugge, L. M., Rennert, C., & Madans, J. H. (1997). The great efficacy of personal and equipment assistance in reducing disability. *American Journal of Public Health*, *87*, 384–392.

White, R. W. (1974). Strategies of adaptation: An attempt at systematic description. In: G. V. Coelho, D. A. Hamburg & J. E. Adams (Eds), *Coping and adaptation* (pp. 47–68). New York: Basic Books.

DISABILITY MEASUREMENT MATRIX: A TOOL FOR THE COORDINATION OF MEASUREMENT PURPOSE AND INSTRUMENT DEVELOPMENT

Barbara M. Altman, Elizabeth K. Rasch and Jennifer H. Madans

ABSTRACT

The multidimensionality of the concept of disability makes the development of questions to measure the concept very complicated. In addition, the purposes of data collection can require a variety of different dimensions of the concept of disability to meet the variety of data uses. This paper proposes a data matrix for use in focusing the methodologist on the issues related to the multidimensionality of the concept and the variety of data needs when planning surveys. Discussions of the three components of the matrix, purpose, conceptual domains and question characteristics, provides the reader with an understanding of the elements of this tool. Multiple tables provide examples of the possible uses of the matrix.

International Views on Disability Measures: Moving Toward Comparative Measurement
Research in Social Science and Disability, Volume 4, 263–284

ISSN: 1479-3547/doi:10.1016/S1479-3547(05)04014-5

The ongoing development of theoretical models of disability has incorporated an ever increasing set of complex concepts and relationships to explain the disabling process (Brandt & Pope, 1997; World Health Organization, 2001). Though disability may appear on the surface to be a simple phenomena, represented for example by a person losing a limb in an auto accident, it turns out to be a mix of interrelated circumstances influenced by the effect the trauma has on the individual, the characteristics of the individual who experiences the health trauma, the characteristics of those around them, the social and structural context they inhabit, the cultural orientation of the community and the policies of the governing bodies. The accident and the resulting impairment are simply what initiates the process.

Recognizing that these interwoven factors contribute to the experience of disability gives some insight into the complications associated with measuring the phenomena. For example, the evaluation of the nature of the trauma takes place initially in a medical setting by medical personnel, so that it can be identified as a crush injury requiring surgical amputation of the left leg, below or above the knee, due to an automobile accident. From the individual's perspective, the physical loss can be identified in several ways, either associated with the pain of the wound, the sense of loss, or the limitation of mobility it imposes. When contextual factors are introduced, including others around the individual, the physical environment and social context (including the culture, the social institutions and established attitudes toward these kinds of problems), multiple layers of meaning (or definition) and a variety of expectations are generated. Those different combinations of circumstance give rise to a variety of ways to view and define the situation which in turn contribute to a variety of ways to measure the outcome which is expressed by the term "disability."

In order to understand and measure this multidimensional and dynamic concept, we need to find a way to examine the relevant characteristics of the individual, the contextual elements and their intersection. We also need to understand the focus or purpose of the measurement as well as the characteristics of the measurement tools (questions, response categories, scaling of questions, mode of delivery and other mundane aspects of the measurement process). To understand how measurement choices impact on the resulting data, we need a tool which at one time can facilitate the examination of the purpose of the data collection, match the aspect of disability that is relevant to that purpose and identify the characteristics of the questions that will tap those aspects of disability within the data collection mode.

THE COMPONENTS OF THE TOOL

Purpose

What is the purpose of the disability data collection exercise or the objectives for including a disability measure in a census or survey? Very often this is not a consideration in the planning of the survey or the development of the measure. However, when faced with a multidimensional concept of this type, it is necessary to clearly understand both the concept and how the data are to be used (what question is being asked) before an appropriate measure can be chosen. In some instances where the concept being measured is less complicated and the purpose of measuring is simple, the variation in the concept can be addressed by providing the range of possibilities in the answer categories. So, for example, the purpose of collecting a demographic characteristic such as marital status, in general, is to be able to track changes in that status or to understand how the variation in that status can influence the social circumstances of the individual, such as income or employment. So, although marital status arrangements have increased in variety it would be relatively simple to provide a list of the major types of relationships in the answer categories to capture a great majority of possibilities. The multidimensionality of the concept of disability however is different than the variety of person A/person B combinations that make up the types of marital statuses. There are more component parts involved in disability and among those component parts much wider variation so that the extent of the possible combinations cannot be captured easily in one set of categorical combinations. Additionally, fulfilling the specific purpose of collecting disability data may require different dimensions of the disability concept thus complicating the measurement process further.

Public policy associated with disability evolved out of concerns about individual and family welfare. As Stone (1979, p. 15) has indicated, all societies have two distributive systems, one based on work and one based on need. When disability evolved as category of need as a 'formal administrative category' (Stone, 1979, p. 27) it provided rights and privileges to a selected group of people. How the category of need was defined became the basis for measurement in the population and the requirement to assess the level of need became the purpose for data collection. Level of need refers to the number who would possibly satisfy the definition of the category and be assumed to need the benefit.

The 'need assessment' purpose has been a driving force in collecting data on disability since disability became a formal administrative category. Very early censuses, for example, counted persons with blindness or deafness ostensibly in order to provide some kinds of services or assistance. In more recent years, additional new uses or purposes for the data have been applied to the disability measures that already are in use in surveys, particularly in health surveys. Limited consideration has been given to the ways that disability were originally defined or to the applicability of those interpretation to the new purposes or uses for the measures. Additionally, even when the purpose of the data is considered in the development of the disability measure, other information needed to meet that purpose is not considered. So, for example, in response to years of concern about restrictions in employment associated with disability, a frequently used question asks about being limited in the kind or amount of work that can be done. Yet, information on the provision of work accommodations, whether the person chooses to work, whether they worked prior to the impairment, what kind of work they are trained for and many other aspects that influence the situation are not obtained. We do not know if persons who do not report work limitations actually have impairments or functional limitations but are well supported by their environment and experience no work limitations. When limitation in work is used as a general measure of disability it distorts conclusions about the employment status and those without disabilities.

With the advent of civil rights legislation related to disability as well as with changing attitudes about what a person with a disability can accomplish, important policy issues require measurement of disability from a radically different approach than one of 'needs assessment.' The needs approach located the policy problem with the individual and their specific lack (of capacity, employment, income, etc.), and sought to understand the types of services required to ameliorate that lack. The focus of a contemporary rights policy perspective is located at the activity level that takes place at the person/environment intersection and seeks to provide data to evaluate how the individual who may have a limitation or impairment is included in social activities. This perspective is termed equalization of opportunity. Concerns about access to education, i.e. are persons with disabilities restricted in the level or type of their educational attainment compared to others, is one example of social inclusion, but any type of participation in activities important at a societal level would be an outcome of concern. Even the employment issue can now be seen from a different perspective, so that while 'needs assessment' was the orientation of the questions about personal limitations in the ability to work and the resulting need for income support, the newer civil rights perspective would ask about how the person's functional limitation interacts with the employment context to either facilitate employment or to make employment difficult. These very different perspectives require different measurement strategies.

Other purposes for which disability data are useful include monitoring of trends in disability as the population ages or as the nation becomes involved in war or as gang violence spreads into various regions of the country. Such trends signal aggregate epidemiological or behavioral changes that can effect building patterns, locations of certain kinds of merchants, need for increased law enforcement or markets for assistive devices. Trend data cumulates information over a period of time, so that it requires consistent measures for a period of years.

Table 1 shows an outline of the major purposes and sub-categories of those purposes that are most commonly found either for nationally representative data or for smaller special projects at the state or organization level. The examples are just a sample of the variety of areas that are relevant within each category of purpose. The important thing to understand is that the purpose sets the framework or perspective from which to view the issues associated with disability measurement. So, for example, the 'needs assessment' perspective focuses on deficits experienced by the person with disability, be they financial or physical, and seeks to identify areas where remedies are needed.

Table 1. Major Purposes, with Examples, of Disability Data Collection Efforts.

Organizing Purpose	Major Categories	Examples
Needs assessment		
	Resource distribution	Income support programs
		Health care programs
	Restoration/control	Rehabilitation programs
		Medical care
	Commerce	Long-term care facilities
		Manufacturers of equipment
Equalization of opportunity		
	Physical access	Housing
		Transportation
	Social access	Education
		Employment
Monitoring trends		
	Demographic relationships	Age, gender, race
	Historical change	Prevalence estimates

Equalization of opportunity purposes seek to evaluate social inclusion and to understand what aspects of the social or physical environment contribute to successful or unsuccessful participation. Separating the orientation of research purpose does not mean purposes are unrelated. The programs developed through needs assessment research can increase opportunities and participation. Finally monitoring trends describes the functioning level of the population as a whole given the programs in place and the characteristics of the population.

Disability Domains

The various conceptual aspects of the disablement process described earlier have been captured in the model developed for the International Classification of Functioning, Disability and Health (ICF). The ICF provides a uniform, standard language and a framework for describing all the dimensions of what is commonly known as disability. In a more detailed way than ever before, it also provides a starting point for considering the relationship of the dimensions to one another. The basic components or parts of the model are grouped in terms of the individual's body functions and structure, individual's activities (from the simplest action to more complicated tasks), individual participation in the social context and the environmental context which reflects both physical and social surroundings of the individual. Using the domains grouped within these four major parts helps with the measurement process because each of the domains can be considered as an element of the process that it is suitable to measure. Each domain, which is identified and defined by the classification, becomes a possible starting point for the operational process which will translate the domain related concepts into observable elements that can be measured. The domains, then, are important elements in the measurement process. However, with so many domains, how do we know which to focus on for our measurement instrument?

The answer to that question lies in the purpose of the measurement or the intended use of the data and how well the various domains of the ICF address that purpose. For example if, from a needs assessment perspective, there was a concern about rehabilitation of persons with missing limbs or the need for limb prostheses, measurement at the body structure/function level would be appropriate. If, however, the needs assessment was concerned about financial support for persons who were unable to find or keep a job, a measure at the participation level of activity would be more relevant. In a similar way, planning for having sufficient long-term care facilities to accommodate the aging baby boomers would be helped by identifying those who need help in doing basic activities such as self-care or basic management of household tasks that are required to remain independent.

Monitoring access to equal opportunity, or the civil rights purpose of measuring disability, requires a different approach. Equal opportunity focuses on the point of interaction between the person and the social context. Equal opportunity refers to having similar choices and expectations as any other person in the social culture, e.g. getting a job, riding on a bus, going to a ball game, or any other form of participation in the society. While it would seem that measurement for this purpose should focus on questions about participation in any or all of these activities, to examine true access, to housing, transportation, employment or any other social role activity, the measurement needs to be at a more basic level of functioning. Identifying those who report inability or limitations to work because of a health problem does not identify those who have health problems, impairments or functional limitations and do not experience that inability or limitation because they have made successful adaptations or accommodations using assistive devices or other tools to allow participation.

Alternatively, measuring at the level of body systems would assume that limitations in these specific forms of function necessarily adversely affect activities and participation when that is not necessarily a one to one relationship. Using the body structure/functioning component of the ICF at this juncture is too detailed for survey measurement, but more importantly does not account for what the integrated person can accomplish by using other areas of functioning to compensate for what is not functional. It is not necessarily the specific impairment itself that is the problem, but the type of functional limitation that it causes in the whole person's abilities which creates the other limitations in activities and participation. If we consider that basic *self initiated* actions, which are influenced in a variety of ways by the numerous types of impairments represented in the body structure/function components of the ICF, are *building blocks* of all activity and subsequent participation, we have a logical starting point for measurement of equalization of opportunity requirements. Those basic self initiated actions include seeing, hearing, walking, communicating, reasoning and of course self-consciousness which to begin with is essential to all of the basic functioning. This list can be expanded to include other specific aspects of self-initiated functioning, such as learning or remembering, which underlay all our actions, activities and ultimate participation. Limitation in any one area can put the person *at risk* for restricted participation, but does not necessarily equate with a restriction.

Measurement at this basic level of action, however, requires that some indication of the participation element of concern be included in the questionnaire as well so that the analysis can be used to answer the question of whether equalization of opportunity has been achieved. If we want to know whether this 'at risk' person, with limitations in one or more basic actions, is employed, we also have to ask some questions about their current employment status. In addition, questions about possible barriers to the form of participation of concern can add further information to subsequent analyses. So, for example, questions about employment will be informed by knowing if the respondent has a car or a useable form of public transportation they can access assuming that such access can facilitate their ability to work.

Table 2 gives a brief outline of the elements of the ICF model, the conceptual areas of the model and a sampling of the domains and categories within those conceptual areas. It also gives examples of operational possibilities for those common categories. We have focused on domains and categories that seem to be more relevant for use in censuses or national health surveys.

Questions Characteristics

The final component of the matrix we are proposing relates to the question design that best operationalizes the categories for the stated purpose of the measurement. Answer categories, for example range from dichotomous, yes/no options to multiple responses that range over levels of severity or some other type of scale. This element of the matrix identifies possible additional information associated with the domains that may or may not be incorporated into the question wording, such as indications of how long the condition has existed. Other elements associated with the organization of the questionnaire, such as the need for skip patterns can also be included in this component of the matrix. Table 3, gives some examples of the question and survey characteristics that are important to the planning process.

THE MATRIX

A basic matrix that connects the purposes for the data collection with the possible domains, helps provide a way to identify the general information needed before undertaking the detailed work of developing the actual questions and answer categories. The idea is to combine the three components described above and configured in Fig. 1, to use as a tool for developing

Table 2. ICF Model Conceptual Components, Sample Domains and Examples of Operational Elements to Represent those Domains.

Conceptual Components	Sample Domains	Elements to be Operationalized
Body functions and structures		
	Global mental functions	Consciousness function – state of awareness and alertness
	Voice and speech functions	Voice functions – function of the production of various sounds by the passage of air through the larynx
	Neuromusculoskeletal and movement related functions	Mobility of joint functions–functions of the range and ease of movement of a joint
Activities and Participation[a]		
Activity	Applying knowledge	Thinking – formulating and manipulating ideas, concepts and images, whether goal oriented or not...
	Mobility	Walking – moving along a surface on foot, step by step, so that one foot is always on the ground.
	Self-care	Washing oneself – washing and drying one's whole body, or body parts, using water and appropriate cleaning and drying materials.
Participation	Mobility	Using transportation – using transportation to move around as a passenger such as being driven in a car or a bus, rickshaw, jitney, animal powered vehicle, or private or public taxi, bus, train, subway, boat or aircraft.
	Domestic life	Acquiring a place to live – buying renting, furnishing and arranging a house, apartment or other dwelling
	Major life areas	Acquiring, keeping and terminating a job – seeking, finding and choosing employment, being hired and accepting employment, maintaining and advancing through a job, trade, occupation or profession and leaving a job in an appropriate manner.
Environmental Factors		
	Products and technology	Products and technology for communication – equipment, products and technologies used by people in activities of sending and

Table 2. *(Continued)*

Conceptual Components	Sample Domains	Elements to be Operationalized
		receiving information, including those adapted or specially designed, located in, on or near the person using them.
	Services, systems and policies	Architecture and construction services, systems and policies – services, systems and policies for the design and construction of buildings, public and private.

[a]Activities and Participation are identified as two separate conceptual areas in the ICF Model, however are combined in the classification scheme due to the overlapping nature of some elements. We have separated them again for clarity and for the purpose of our discussion which is based more on the theoretical model.

Table 3. Question Characteristics, Survey Characteristics and Other Methodological Characteristics to Consider.

Methodological Components	Elements	Example
Question characteristics		
	Introduction – cause, duration	Because of a physical, mental or emotional health problem lasting 6 months or more
	Answer categories	Yes/no; severity scale
	Need for a standard reference	Is there a standard against which a respondent will be compared – often a standard is assumed and not specified
	Capacity or performance	Is the question framed to focus on what a person does or what they are capable of doing?
	Question language	Avoid negative language
Survey characteristics		
	Space limitations	Survey length and other elements allow for how much time to focus on this topic
	Skip pattern	Does space and time restraints require a skip pattern
	Screener	If time and space requirements are severe, sometimes a screener is necessary to identify who will answer the disability questions. This screener then becomes a key to everything that follows

Table 3. *(Continued)*

Methodological Components	Elements	Example
	Mode	Mailed questionnaires need to be simpler and more straight forward than in person interviews.

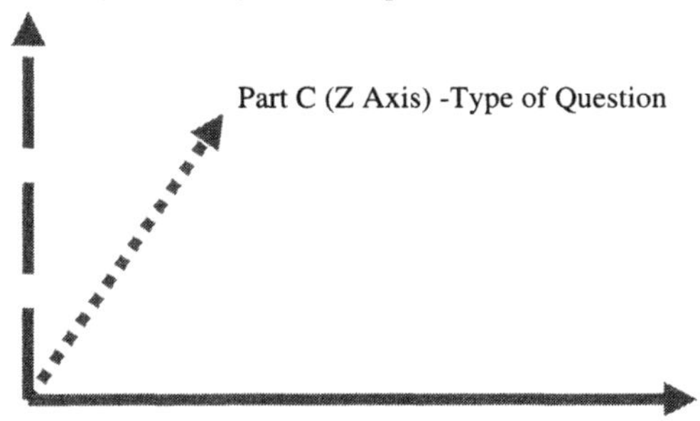

Fig. 1. Dimensions of Disability Measurement Matrix.

operational concepts to satisfy the purpose of measurement. Part A, the primary purpose of the data collection is the dominant element in this matrix since the other two elements are chosen to satisfy that purpose.

The Disability Measurement Matrix clarifies the relationships between measurement purpose, disability conceptualization and characteristics of the measurement instrument. This matrix *does not* work as a selection tool that will provide actual questions. Rather it should be seen as a tool to help the researcher to think through, in structured steps, the development of their disability measurement. First the purpose of the data collection needs to be examined and understood. Once that is established, the relative domains of the disability process can be identified. There may be numerous domains that are appropriate, but constraints of the data collection mode come into play to set limits on the number and type of domains that can be used. The process may require a few iterations to get the pieces to fit together well, each iteration refining the product further. Additionally, we recognize that specific purposes of measurement can be addressed by different conceptual elements of the ICF model or of other multi-dimensional disability models.[1] Therefore the disability measurement matrix was developed to delineate the association between measurement purposes, measurement concepts and characteristics of questions that best reflect the concepts. However, since the ICF is attempting to standardize language and since it is the most comprehensive model available today we recommend its use.

To illustrate the functioning of the matrix as a tool, we have created four additional tables to show the matrix in use. These tables are a result of the Washington Group activities to develop general measures of disability for use in censuses and reflect the work presented at the second meeting of the Washington Group in Ottawa, Canada (see Washington Group website at http://www.cdc.gov/nchs/citygroup.htm for more information on that meeting and other Washington Group activities).

Table 4–6 demonstrate working with the three major purposes of measurement, Part A, and the four major components of disability (as defined by the ICF), Part B. The four components and some of the sub-domains are captured across the top of the table and the measurement purposes are identified down the left side of the table. Each of these tables show examples of the three different general purposes discussed earlier. In some cases, a particular topic may appear in all three of the purpose areas. That is because a topic, such as medical care can be approached from several perspectives, either as a program that provides services to a particular population or as a form of participation in the social structure. Obviously we can monitor trends of almost anything, so medical care could have been included under that purpose as well in the form of monitoring use of medical services by the population of concern.

Table 4 is a working example of a matrix focusing on a set of 'needs assessment' purposes. The general domains of the ICF are captured across the top of the table and the sample purposes are identified down the left side of the table. The Environmental domain is identified by two sub-categories, the environment in general and the specific environmental element associated with assistive devices. Assistive devices were included in this way because of their extremely important function in helping the individual navigate the environment and their role in moderating limitations. Use of assistive devices is a domain that probably should be considered in any measurement of disability. In the same way, the Activity domain is divided into basic functioning or actions and a more general approach to activity. Finally, participation and body structure/function are represented.

To use the table, identify the purpose for data collection and analysis. Using the first purpose listed in Table 4 as an example, consider the possibilities offered by each domain for the measurement of relevant aspects of disability. If we are concerned about collecting data for assessing the needs for personal assistant services, the description of the general environment will give valuable information on the context in which the personal assistance will take place and the knowledge about the assistive device use or needs will provide valuable information about what the individual has or needs to function in that environment. Participation, in this type of data collection will either reflect what the individual does on a regular basis, or the kinds of participation the individual would like to do with the help of a personal assistant. General measures of activity, such as tasks associated with independence would give a picture of what the person in question is capable of accomplishing themselves and what basic activities require assistance. Information on basic functioning in this context will give a better picture of the exact limitations which create the other problems in activity and participation. In a data collection process that is limited by time or space, this information is probably the most basic. Finally, information on the nature of the impairment will inform the nature of the basic limitations so, for example, knowing that paralysis is the cause of lack of mobility rather than a missing limb sheds light on the detailed nature of the types of personal assistance that may be required.

Table 5 focuses on equalization of opportunity purposes using the same categories of question domains as outlined in Table 4. The interpretation of the conceptual domains for this purpose have a different orientation than those associated for 'needs assessment' particularly in the areas of activity and participation, although the conceptual components associated with environment may overlap. The differences in approach are most easily comprehended for the specific purpose of collecting data to understand employment. In a 'needs assessment' approach, we ask about persons with limitations in or an inability to work because of the health problem, mental, physical or emotional. That measure gives us an idea of the group who will probably need some kind of support through disability benefits to supplement their income. However, in an 'equal opportunity' approach, we ideally want to identify anyone who has a functioning limitation, either sensory, physical or mental limitation, which could in some way interfere with working. For this purpose the identification of the functioning limitation is separated from the question about working in order to be able to capture not only those who find that functioning limitations preclude working, but to be able to identify those who while they report functioning limitation report no limitations in work or employment. In a similar way, comparison between the purpose of understanding access to medical care (and equalization of opportunity purpose) and understanding the needs for medical rehabilitation (a needs assessment purpose) one can see that the orientation

Table 4. First Step Examination of Purpose and Conceptual Domains of Measurement – Needs Assessment Disability Measurement Matrix.

Part A	Part B: Question Concepts Associated with Measurement of Disability for a Variety of Purposes					
Purpose of Measurement	Environment		Participation	Activity		Body Structure and Function
	General	Assistive Devices		General	Basic Function	Impairment
Part I: Needs assessment	Focus of data collection *is on the individual* who will be served by the program or product					
Service provision product development	Organization focus is a key to defining what is measured. Data needs for individual data are really organization specific. Long-term care provision vs. advocacy for employment directs the focus of questions into very different areas. Does the service provision single out one or several types of conditions, i.e. developmental disabilities or paralysis, or are the services or products necessary for one or more individuals					
1. Personal assistant services	What are physical or other environmental barriers to be overcome	Are devices available and are they needed	Where does help need to take place – home/work or other	Type of personal assistance. Needed-bathing, etc.	Limited mobility/ difficulty making decisions	Paralysis or cognitive, etc.
2. Device manufacturer	Where will device be used	What is already available	Where/how will item be used	What task process needs to be facilitated, for example – driving a car	Nature of necessary functioning compensation	Nature of orientation of substitution. For example – site where prostheses is needed
3. Advocacy services	What are the advocacy issues are they associated with building structure	How can access to devices be implemented	What forms of participation sought	The nature of the abilities and limitations needs to be known in order to facilitate the advocates negotiation for specific needs		

Purpose of Measurement	Environment	Assistive Devices	Participation	Activity	Basic Function	Impairment
4. Rehabilitation	Rehabilitation is a commonly used type of service that generally focuses on restoring some function. Understanding the client's context as well as their abilities and limitations should help understanding the nature of the function that needs to be restored.					
(a) Education programs	What are environmental barriers that prevent access of potential clients	Use as well as need for devices	What outcome is program seeking, employment? or other? What is the participation deficit that needs correction?	Focus of education programs mainly on learning, so these two measures would only be relevant to areas that can be taught within context of program. So if self-help skills are a focus of program, self-help skills should be measured.		What is the source of problem, sensory or mental or physical useful for directing funding requests
(b) Medical rehabilitation (services)	What are environmental barriers that prevent access of potential clients	Matching of assistive device to individual needs	What is the participation deficit that Medical Rehabilitation can address	Self-help skills – inventory to locate deficits	Improved capacity will contribute to basic functioning	What is the specific body structure that needs attention

Table 5. First Step: Examination of Purpose and Conceptual Domains of Measurement – Equalization of Opportunity.

Part A	Part B: Question Concepts Associated with Measurement of Disability for a Variety of Purposes					
Purpose of Measurement	Environment		Participation	Activity		Body Structure and Function
	General	Assistive Device		General	Basic Functioning	Impairment
Part II: Equalization of opportunity	Focus of data collection ***is upon the complete population*** that will be benefited by civil rights legislation. Equalization in this context can involve development of programs such as those indicated above to improve participation access. Measurement in this context is very closely associated with understanding the population at risk of experiencing restrictions, discrimination or problems with access					
Policy/program development for population groups	Policy and program in this context refers to the development of national or state policy to address problem areas, provide support for development of general access or mandate civil rights. Understanding the general circumstances of persons similar in some basic ways allows legislative initiatives to generate laws or programs to benefit large groups of individuals rather than just one.					
1. Americans with Disabilities Act (ADA) Implementation – directed toward improved participation	Identification of environmental barriers that exist for all types of limitations	Use of assistive devices represents forms of accommodations	Since ADA guarantees participation this is an essential component of measure, but one that everyone should be asked of	Identification of limitations in basic tasks can provide insight into why a person identified with functioning limitations experiences participation restriction – an intervening variable	Identification of sensory, cognitive and physical functioning limitations identifies persons 'at risk' of participation restriction – a key indicator for this purpose	While the ADA definition is based on impairments,[a] impairments do not provide the level of functioning which is the essential building block to serve this purpose

Purpose of Measurement	Environment	Assistive Device	Participation	Activity	Basic Functioning	Impairment
2. Employment	Identification of environmental barriers in transportation and at employment sites	Are assistive devices available or needed	Major role participation is the concern here, not the limitation in participation, but whether or not the person is actually involved in the role	Ability to do tasks relevant to type of employment. An intervening variable as indicated above	Identification of sensory, cognitive, mental health or physical functioning known to be 'a risk factor' for work limitations	Not particularly relevant to measuring to facilitate participation
3. Long-term care	Identification of home barriers that prevent independent living	Assistive device use masks level of care need has to be included	Participation relevant to this purpose more limited to reflecting basic levels of involvement in home	Self care and independence limitations are key elements of cause for support needs	Functioning is more important than impairment here – it is central to the ability to maintain independence	Identification of the type of impairment is useful to indicate type of long term care needed
4. Medical care (access)	Identification of possible barriers that can prevent accessing office, hospital or other facility	Availability of assistive devices on site such as mobility devices	Participation of relevance here is in some form of insurance plan	Types of activities concern use of and access to transportation, arranging appointments	Basic functioning related to do activities necessary to make and keep appointments	Nature of impairment not relevant to getting access to medical care

[a]ADA defines disability as one of the following: (1) having a physical or mental impairment that substantially limits one or more of the major life activities of such individual; (2) a record of such impairment; (3) or being regarded as having such an impairment (Sec. 3(2), 42U.S.C. 12102, 1990).

Table 6. First Step: Examination of Purpose and Conceptual Domains of Measurement – Trend Monitoring.

Part A	Part B: Question Concepts Associated with Measurement of Disability for a Variety of Purposes					
Purpose of Measurement	Environment		Participation	Activity		Body Structure and Function
	General	Assistive Device		General	Function	Impairment
Part III: Trend monitoring	Focus of this process is to identify, in the aggregate population, changes in prevalence rates of a particular indicator that reflects policy concerns. Used in research on the size and characteristics of selected populations, changes in geographic distribution of those populations					
1. Prevalence rates	Identifying geographic and structural barriers experienced will provide context of other variables	Identifying all users of assistive devices will provide use prevalence, does not address need	Identifying a form of participation limitations will provide population with that limitation only, not those with potential to have that limitation	Identifying activity limitations will provide population who have problems with specific activities or actions not those with potential to have those problems	Identifying all types of functional limitations will provide the population at risk for activity and participation limitation	Identifying any impairments will provide the population with specific impairments – useful for epidemiological research
2. Trends	Trend analysis requires that prevalence data be repeated in the exact same format over the required time period. Changes in measurement over the short-term limit the development of trend data.					

of the use of the data collection can be very different for areas that might be deemed to be very similar. Questioning about access to medical care (equalization of opportunity) would be formatted in a way similar to the employment example above. The questions about functioning would be separated from questions about the use of medical services. For a 'needs assessment' approach, the connection of the functioning problem to the health care need has to be made within the same questions such that a respondent is asked 'because of a physical, mental or emotional health problem, do you need physical or mental health therapy?' In the first example where the questions are separate, we would know what proportion of the population with the specified limitations uses some specified health care professional. We would not be able to identify those who need such care but do not receive it without asking further questions. In the second, 'needs assessment' approach, we would possibly identify most of the persons with limitations who need some form of therapy. However, without asking further questions, we would not know who receives the therapy and how much and who does not receive any at all.

Estimates and monitoring of prevalence rates generally focus on the level of functioning in the population. Interest is usually in the percentage of the total population that experience limitations in activities or participation, but it can relate to use of devices or environmental characteristics. Differences among populations and also population subgroups can be monitored as well. Table 6 examines the type of conceptualizations that might be associated with monitoring trends. It is particularly important to specify the characteristics being monitored to understand what the trends are demonstrating. So, for example, if the analyst documents the number of persons who report limitations in ability to work, they are identifying a sub-population of persons with disabilities who actually experience a work limitation associated with whatever functional limitations they also experience. This measure will not reflect the employment rate of the population with functional limitations which requires identifying persons with a broad range of functional limitations (sensory, mobility, communication, etc.) and examining actual employment among those with and without these functional limitations. The trends in these two different measures are related conceptually and empirically different.

In Table 7, we show the addition of the third component, question and mode characteristics, to the matrix. The purpose of the data collection and the selected domain are found in the left hand columns of the table and the characteristics of the questions and other methodological issues are distributed across the column heads. This table assumes that multiple domains

Table 7. Second Step – Examining the Purpose and Operationalized Domain for Methodological Issues.

	Part C: Question Characteristics for Use with Specific Purposes and Domains of Disability						
Part A: Purpose of Measurement	Duration	Capacity Performance	Severity	Cause	Need for Standard Reference	No. of Answer Categories	Type of Problem
Service provision product development	Organization focus is a key to defining what is measured. Data needs are organization-specific. LTC provision vs. advocacy for employment directs focus of questions into very different areas. Does the service provision single out one or several types of conditions, i.e. developmental disabilities or paralysis						
1. Personal assistant services	Duration of problem to this point may not be necessary information, but expected duration may be necessary	Questions should focus on what a person is able to do in this context – performance, not their abilities in an ideal situation	Severity of problem is a key to understanding the types and frequency of the services requires	Cause of problem may help direct service needs to an agency specializing in that condition or problem	What is the comparison standard – other people the same age, other people with the same condition? Some hypothetical norm?	Depends on the detail necessary	Specific details of PA would need to assist with may help matching client and service provider
2. Education programs	Duration may be useful to understand level of educational needs	Information on capacity if available could facilitate planning program	Severity of problem useful to developing program	Cause very necessary to identify developmental problems from purely physical may relate to eligibility	Standard reference could be level of ability at beginning of program – useful for evaluation	Depends on questions asked. Measures of severity need multiple categories of answers	Related in this context to capacity – helps focus program planning

Equalization of opportunity	Equalization refers to development of techniques, processes and systems of service provision which facilitate equal access to all types of social participation. Focus is on type of service that can provide equal access.						
1. Employment	Duration of employment limitation may provide clue as how old skills are	Performance now is useful information for what accommodations may be needed	Severity of functional limitations could inform analysis	On the face, cause of limitation does not seem essential	Need for standard reference probably useful for comparisons	Multiple categories generally provides more information, depends on time and space constraints	Type of problem may shed light on solutions – e.g. if problem is transportation rather than anything else
2. Education programs	Conditions of longer duration may be a factor in access – could be an important analytic variable	What is performance level – may influence continuation in program or access to another	Used to distribute resources, more severe problems require greater resources	Cause not necessary relevant here	Need for standard reference probably useful for comparisons	For purposes of providing individual services, more detail is useful	Same as above and if it differs from cause, is added information for planning

have been selected for measurement and shows some of the differences between data collection for needs assessment for service provision or for examining equalization of opportunity. Each of the methodological elements should be considered within the context of the domain selected and the established purpose. We have included one domain for each purpose as an example, but multiple domains can be considered in turn.

DISCUSSION AND CONCLUSION

The disability matrix is proposed as a tool to guide the thinking process when developing appropriate disability measures for use in survey's and censuses. It allows survey planners to orient their consideration of possible ways to operationalize the components of disability by focusing first on the purpose of data collection and then selecting relevant domains of measurement. A very important contribution of the matrix is the way it demonstrates how operationalizing measurement in a specific element of one domain of the classification narrows the conceptualization of disability being used.

NOTES

1. The ICF includes multiple conceptual elements such as body structures, body functions, activities and participation, and environmental and personal factors. Other models, such as the IOM or Nagi model, include somewhat different conceptual elements such as health conditions (pathology), impairments, functional limitations, activity limitations, and the physical/psychosocial environment.

REFERENCE

Brandt, A., & Pope, D. (1997). *Enabling America: Assessing the role of rehabilitation science and engineering*. Washington, DC: National Academy Press.

Stone, D. A. (1979). *The disabled state*. Philadelphia, PA: Temple University Press.

World Health Organization. (2001). *International classification of functioning, disability and health*. WHO: Geneva, Switzerland.

ABOUT THE AUTHORS

Barbara M. Altman, a sociologist with a Ph.D. from the University of Maryland is currently a special assistant on Disability Statistics at the National Center for Health Statistics and an adjunct associate professor at the University of Maryland, College Park. She is currently involved in revision of the measures of disability in the American Community Survey and has a key role in the Washington Group, an international group seeking to develop culturally compatible measures of disability worldwide. Her disability research interests focus in three areas: disability definition and measurement in survey data; access to, financing and utilization of health care services by persons with disabilities, particularly working-age persons and women with disabilities; and disability among minority groups. She is the author of numerous articles and book chapters on disability topics, and she is currently co-editor of the series *Research in Social Science and Disability*.

Yerker Andersson, Ph.D. is a professor emeritus of sociology at Gallaudet University. He has also developed a program in the new field of study, Deaf Studies. He is a former co-chair of the American Sociological Association Committee on Society and Persons with Disabilities. He has presented papers on the sociological aspects of deaf people widely in the world. He is a former president and now an honorary member of the World Federation of the Deaf. Appointed by President Clinton with the consent by the US Senate, he has served on the National Council on Disability. He is a former member of the US-sponsored international committee on disability tabulations, known as DIST AB.

Sharon N. Barnartt, Ph.D., is professor of sociology at Gallaudet University. She has co-authored two books: Deaf President Now: The 1988 Revolution at Gallaudet University (1995) and Contentious Politics in the Disability and Deaf Communities (2001). She has also presented papers and published widely in the areas of socio-economic status and disability/deafness, legal and disability policy issues, and social movements in the deaf and disability communities. She is a former president of the Society for

Disability Studies, co-editor of Research in Social Science and Disability and on the editorial board of *Journal of Disability Policy Studies*.

Alicia Bercovich is a demographer with a Ph.D. in social sciences and M.Sc. in mathematics. She is the coordinator of the Population Census Committee at the Brazilian Bureau of the Census (IBGE) since 1997. She also coordinates the participation of Brazil in the Joint Population Census for the Mercosur Countries, Bolivia and Chile and is a member of the Steering Committee of the Washington Group on Disability Statistics.

She was head of the IBGE Population Division (1991–1994), head of the Research and Data Preparation Division for the 1980 Census, and visiting scholar at the Population Research Center, of the University of Texas at Austin. She has published several papers, chapters, and reports on demographic topics, especially on demographic discontinuities; the youth wave and its impact on the labor market; fertility and race; and the demography of violence.

Ken Black is an assistant director in the Health and Disability Section of the Australian Bureau of Statistics (ABS). He has been with the ABS for 20 years – with a period from 1993 till 1999 with the Australian Institute of Health and Welfare – and has worked closely with disability issues including the 1993, 1998, and 2003 Surveys of Disability, Ageing, and Carers, development and testing of disability modules for inclusion in non-disability-specific household surveys, the successful development and testing of a disability-related 'core activity, need for assistance' question set for inclusion in the Australian 2006 National Census of Population and housing, and provision of assistance to countries in the Asia Pacific region relating to the collection and dissemination of data on people with a disability.

Roberta Crialesi, M.A., is head of Health Statistics Section at the Italian National Institute of Statistics where she is responsible for several epidemiological surveys relating to abortions, miscarriages, notification of infectious diseases, as well as cause of death. She is also involved in hospital statistics covering patients treated, hospital infrastructure and resources. In this field she has initiated a number of innovative projects aimed at improving the quality and dissemination of health and health-related information. She also has a long experience with large-scale surveys with emphasis on health interview surveys. Besides survey methods, her current research interests focus on different topics such as inequality in health, morbidity and disability, aging, and quality of survival. She has been a consultant and has participated in many expert meetings at the national and international level. She is a member of the Washington Group on Disability Statistics.

Elena De Palma is a senior researcher at the Italian National Institute of Statistics (Istat), Unit of Health Statistics Service. She is involved in the development of the "Statistical Information System on Disability" project, promoted by the Italian Minister of Welfare. She was a member of the Planning Committee for the 3rd meeting of the Washington Group on Disability Statistics. Her main contributions to Washington Group activities include studies entitled: "Comparative analysis of general measure(s) on disability used in Europe" and "Comparative analysis of Minimum European Health Module and Questions Used in Europe." She is also member of the Istat working group on the survey on disability and health services.

Arne H. Eide, Ph.D. (social psychology), is research director at SINTEF Health Research and professor in Rehabilitation at Sør-Trøndelag University College. His background is from health and social policy and social psychology, with behavior research as speciality. He has extensive international experience from research in the fields of disability and rehabilitation.

Nora Groce, Ph.D., is an associate professor in the Division of Global Health, Yale School of Public Health. Dr. Groce is a medical anthropologist, interested in the area of global health and international development with particular emphasis on cross-cultural systems of health care and health as human rights issues. Her research interests include issues of disability in international health and development, violence as a global public health problem and equity in access to health care in ethnic and minority communities. She is director of the Yale/WHO Collaborating Center and Co-Chair of the Disability Studies Group at the Yale Institute of Social and Policy Studies and holds a joint appointment in the Yale Department of Anthropology and Yale Institute for Social and Policy Studies. She serves regularly as an advisor to UN agencies such as WHO, UNICEF, as well as to a number of non-governmental organizations.

Gerry E. Hendershot was trained in sociology and demography at the University of Michigan and the University of Chicago. After serving on the faculties of several colleges and universities, including Vanderbilt University and Brown University, he joined the federal government in 1976 and served as a supervisory health statistician at the National Center for Health

Statistics until 2001. He is the author of more than 40 scientific publications on disability and other public health topics. He is now a private consultant on projects related to disability and health statistics.

Mitchell E. Loeb, M.Sc. (Epidemiology), is a researcher at SINTEF Health Research. He has over 25 years of experience in epidemiological research methodology and the analysis of statistical research data. In recent years his efforts have concentrated on the field of disability research in particular in the setting of low-income countries of southern Africa.

Jennifer H. Madans is currently associate director for Science, National Center for Health Statistics (NCHS). In this capacity, she is responsible for planning and developing NCHS's data collection and analysis programs. Dr. Madans began her career at NCHS in 1978 and has served as acting director of the Division of Analysis, director of the Division of Epidemiology, and deputy director of the Center. She directed two of NCHS's earliest and largest national longitudinal studies, the NHANES I Epidemiologic Follow-up Study and the National Nursing Home Survey Follow-up. These surveys initiated a major redirection of NCHS survey programs. She also directed the major redesign of the National Health Interview Study. She is a fellow of the American Statistical Association.

Ros Madden has led the disability statistics work program at the Australian Institute of Health and Welfare (AIHW) since 1992. Her unit has published a range of population data analyses including: a series of AIHW reports on definition and prevalence of different disabilities; reports on disability and aging, disability and related factors (exploring the International Classification of Functioning, Disability, and Health (ICF) model statistically), children's disability; and three reports, commissioned by Australian disability administrators, on unmet need for disability support services. Administrative data are the key aspects of the work, and the unit works in partnership with Commonwealth, State, and Territory governments on a number of disability and health-related data collections. Ros and her unit anchor the AIHW international work with the World Health Organization on the ICF.

Margaret Mbogoni is a statistician in the Demographic and Social Statistics Branch at the United Nations Statistics Division. Her main area of work is development and review of population and housing census methodology, including the development of international guidelines to be used by countries during the next round of censuses. She has also worked extensively in the area of disability statistics including contributing to the development of the WHO ICF as well as the United Nations Guidelines and Principles for the Development of Disability Statistics. She is also involved in providing technical assistance, through conducting workshops, to countries to improve their capacity to produce and disseminate accurate and relevant statistics. Ms. Mbogoni holds a Ph.D. in demography from the University of Pennsylvania, USA and a B.A. in sociology from Makerere University, Uganda.

Angela Me is currently the chief of the Social and Demographic Statistics Section in the Statistical Division of the UNECE. Her main areas of responsibility include population and housing census, health statistics, migration statistics, gender statistics, and statistics related to the monitoring of the Millennium Development Goals. In her previous job, at the UNSD, she also worked in the area of disability statistics where she assisted countries to strengthen their capacity to collect and disseminate disability statistics. Ms. Me holds a Ph.D. in Statistics from the University of Padua and a Master in Statistics and Demography from the same University.

Helen Namirembe-Nviiri is a principal statistician working with the Uganda Bureau of Statistics. She is currently heading the Population Statistics Section under the Directorate of Population and Social Statistics. At the same time she is working on the 2002 Uganda Population and Housing Census as Deputy Technical Officer. She has seven years of experience on household surveys, which include the 2000/2001 Demographic and Health Survey and the Uganda National Household Surveys (Income and Expenditure surveys). She has participated in the design of census and survey instruments, which have included questions on disability statistics. Particularly, she has drafted instruction guidelines for the questionnaires that include disability concepts and definitions and she has also participated in the training of field interviewers. The knowledge gained from the UN Disability workshop for Africa Region held in September 2001 in Uganda, and her participation in the Washington City Group meetings on Disability have led to tremendous improvement in the area of disability measurement in Uganda.

Elizabeth K. Rasch, MS, PT, is an associate service fellow at the National Center for Health Statistics, CDC, working in the area of disability statistics. She is a Ph.D. candidate at the University of Maryland, Department of Physical Therapy and Rehabilitation Science, with a concentration in Epidemiology. Her research interests include the health of persons with disabilities, factors that contribute to disability, as well as the use of and access to healthcare services by persons with disabilities. Her dissertation focuses on the incidence and consequences of secondary health conditions in persons with mobility limitations. She has been actively involved in research since 1985 and has published articles and book chapters on topics related to disability and rehabilitation.

www.ingramcontent.com/pod-product-compliance
Ingram Content Group UK Ltd.
Pitfield, Milton Keynes, MK11 3LW, UK
UKHW020845290926
15470UKWH00004B/1554

9 780762 312825